The Adventurous
Couple's Guide
to Strap-On Sex

The Adventurous Couple's Guide to Strap-On Sex

Violet Blue

CLEIS
PRESS

Published in the United States by Cleis Press Inc.,
P.O. Box 14697, San Francisco, California 94114.

Printed in the United States.
Cover design: Scott Idleman
Cover photograph: Marin/Getty Images
Book design: Karen Quigg
Cleis Press logo art: Juana Alicia
First Edition.
10 9 8 7 6 5 4

Library of Congress Cataloging-in-Publication Data

Blue, Violet.
      The Adventurous couple's guide to strap-on sex /
Violet Blue—1st edition.
            p. cm.
      ISBN 978-1-57344-278-7 (pbk. : alk. paper)
      1. Sex instruction. 2. Sex. 3. Sex toys. 4. Sexual
excitement. I. Title.

      HQ31.B575 2007
      613.9'6—dc22

                              2007015736

Acknowledgments

As always, admiration and friendship go to Frédérique Delacoste and Felice Newman; our relationships mean more than I can express here. My deepest feelings are reserved for my family—Survival Research Laboratories and Mark Pauline. My love belongs to Jonathan. For fun, for love, for mischief: Hacker Boy.

Contents

Chapter 1

The Forbidden Zone

Strap-on play for couples means many things to many couples—but primarily, when we think of a girl and a boy and their strap-on, we have visions of "bend over boyfriend" in our heads. That's not to say that this sublime sex act is all a couple might do with a sexy harness and perky dildo. It's perhaps the main event (and the headlining act of this book), but couples can employ strap-ons whenever they want an extra, always-hard cock ready for action. He might wear it for her in addition to his own for double the pleasure, or when he needs a breather but she's primed for action. She can certainly give him the anal attention he deserves, or she may just make him into a Blowjob Betty for a session or two. And together they can employ a strap-on with a friend, for play with another guy (three dicks, no waiting) or a friendly female third.

But for most couples, finding information about using strap-ons for pegging (male anal penetration) is scarce, out of date, or lumped together with other sex acts so as not to be too overt about what's really going on—women strapping it on and

giving it to the guys. The truth is, it's all about male anal pleasure and eroticism, on the receiving end of a woman's (silicone)
cock. For lovers who understand this, there is much power and
joy to be found in the forbidden zone.

Women, Men and Strap-Ons

Give a man the anal attention he craves, and you might as well
have tossed a pat of butter into a hot pan. Even the hint of anal
stimulation during sex may send a warm rush across his body
from toes to fingertips, set him swooning in response to your
attentions, and ignite a powerful arousal, from cock to heart
to head in an explosive instant. Anal stimulation can be like hit-
ting a pleasure switch—even the lightest touch on the outside
of the anus can sweep him straight to orgasm.

To me, the discovery that a male lover enjoys receiving anal
penetration opens up a whole world of sexual adventure
between the two of us. It means that he wants to share something really intimate—and something he finds powerfully
pleasurable—with me. I know that he probably hasn't been able
to play like this with most of his other lovers (although, as I
explain later, straight couples have taken over the male anal fron-
tier), but he feels confident that we can do it, and do it lustily
enough to make us both satisfied. When a man tells me he wants
me to strap it on and give it to him—I know I've found a lover
who is playful, trusting, interested in having excellent sexual
communication, and who thinks I'm the hottest girl for the job.
Penetration is one of those very amazing things that connect
you with him like nothing else, and it can be an incredible turn-
on for both of you. With your finger or fingers, a dildo, or a

vibrator, you enter into a realm of pleasure that is as deep for him as it is intimate for both of you.

Sometimes it's just the idea of strap-on sex that's enough to set your fantasies in motion. Wearing a strap-on dildo, even if you don't do anything with it, makes for a sexual encounter like no other, especially if you've never tried it and he's never seen you in one. It's a sensation full of revelations and sexual giddiness that must be experienced to be understood. For starters, there's the incredible arousal that usually comes with playing with "your dick." Perhaps you're turning the tables on your lover, strapping on a sexy black harness and fastening in a dildo to jut jauntily from between your legs.

Will you follow through with everything your new dick implies? And what would that entail, exactly; strutting around in a pair of high heels, or going all the way and dressing extrabutch in a tank top and work boots? See how hot and bothered you get while stroking your new erect appendage, pretending to jack off. With a strap-on cock, you can even rub it all over your lover's face and ask for a blowjob. Ultimately, you can take total control and penetrate him, giving you something you want, and him something he needs.

> Sometimes it's just the idea of strap-on sex that's enough to set your fantasies in motion.

Sound hot? It is. Being on either side of a strap-on can be equally arousing and sexually satisfying for both participants. Many men find that a dildo stimulates their anus and prostate in unspeakably pleasurable ways, while women who strap it on often find that the strap-on itself can bring them to orgasm through pressure from the dildo's base—not to mention the

benefits of supplemental toys such as strap-in dildos and
wearable clit vibes. Whether it's a power exchange fantasy, a
gender-bending scenario or just the blissful sensation of being
inside your lover—or for him, feeling your lover inside you—
few thrills can compare to strap-on sex. Best of all, there are
no consequences to strap-on play, unless you consider increased
intimacy a risk. Being penetrated and played with by a lover in
a harness is just as fun, intense and sexually exciting as doing
the strapping, and the orgasmic potential is eye opening.

The *Bend Over Boyfriend* (Pegging) Phenom

Obviously, men have been enjoying anal pleasure since time
began—if there's something that feels good to play with, you
better bet primates will see how much fun they can have with
it. However, that doesn't mean that straight men playing with
their butts—and asking their female partners to join in the fun—
was instantly socially acceptable. When porn was in its infancy,
only on rare occasions would viewers see such a "taboo" sex act
on-screen, and this antiquated attitude toward this sex act continues in mainstream porn to this day. Only in the "golden age"
of porn in the 1970s and '80s did we start to see hints of the
hotness of women strapping it on and giving it to the guys, in
films such as *Myra Breckenridge* (1970), *Score* (1973) and *The Opening
of Misty Beethoven* (1976). But these glimpses were sadly rare, if
titillating as all get-out when they happened.

But then in the 1990s a funny thing happened. Women-owned
sex toy retailer Good Vibrations noticed that more and more,
straight couples were buying strap-ons and dildos to use with
each other—not to give to their lesbian friends as Hanukkah

gifts. And they were excited about it—and craving as much information about their intended, potential sex act as they could find.

The sex educator on staff (namely Dr. Carol Queen) connected with a lesbian porn filmmaking company, and came up with a plan to make a how-to video for straight couples about male anal penetration. Thus the video *Bend Over Boyfriend* and the eponymous term for the sex act were created in one swift stroke, and the video sold (and continues to sell) like hotcakes. The *Bend Over Boyfriend* phenomenon brought on by the how-to video of the same name (fatalemedia.com) has skyrocketed harness and dildo sales to heterosexual couples across the nation.

A few years later, in June 2001, popular national sex columnist Dan Savage opened a contest to readers of his column asking for suggestions of a common name for the sex act. The term "bend over boyfriend" was in widespread use as a catchall for the video, the video genre and the act, due to the video's popularity, and perhaps Savage tapped into the general vibe that such a long and clumsy phrase missed the immediacy required in sex slang linguistics. One could certainly say, "I want to blow you" or "felching is gross," but substituting "bend over boyfriend" in place of "blow" or "felch" wouldn't make your English professor happy, nor your Craigslist ad successful. Savage received 12,103 responses to the naming quandary, with three main contenders for the title: "BOB," for the *Bend Over Boyfriend* video and phrase (2,721 votes), "punt" as in kicking one's ball to the opposing team (4,166 votes), and "peg" for its many evocative definitions (the winner, at 5,216 votes).

Pegging is male-penetrative anal sex for straight couples, and essential to its eroticism for participants is the emphasis placed on gender in this heterosexual exchange. Past conventional wisdom on the subject of anal sex (and I think there is such a thing), suggests that anal is only loved and practiced by gay guys and really bad girls. Not so anymore. Perhaps the fact that straight men are interested in receptive anal exploration with their female partners comes from increased awareness about prostate pleasure—with the prostate sometimes being called "the male G-spot." Or maybe men today are just more comfortable and confident about their sexuality and can see through all the contrived myths linking male anal sex and homosexuality to make up their own minds (because not all gay men like anal sex, and being penetrated can't *make* someone gay no matter how much they might want it to). But most likely, because our culture talks about sex more than ever before, happy, horny and adventurous guys and gals are looking at each other's bodies as the pleasure playgrounds they were meant to be. And that's a *really* good thing.

> Pegging is male-penetrative anal sex for straight couples, and essential to its eroticism for participants is the emphasis placed on gender in this heterosexual exchange.

As a sex act, straight couples playing with strap-ons has proven itself to be a very lucrative and popular emerging (and exciting) area of sexual expression. Lucrative, that is, for those toy companies savvy enough to understand what's at play here; the *Bend Over Boyfriend* phenom has befuddled the more traditional sex toy retailers and porn directors, and also sex advice authors and porn reviewers of all orientations. As noted sexologist Dr. Carol Queen said in the introduction to *Bend Over Boyfriend*, "Straight couples are reinventing anal sex." Because even if uptight porn directors and novelty manufacturers may not have the faintest idea why a couple buys a harness, we can be pretty certain that they're doing it because it's *fun*.

Chapter 2

What It Isn't

E ven though the couples doing it are pretty clear about where they stand with the pleasures of plundering the male back door, some people still have distinct discomfort about what it all might mean. My belief is that this is an expression of homo-phobia, projected and internalized, even though this is strictly a straight sex act. For instance, in most every mainstream sex guide you pick up, if you can find a reference to the prostate gland at all (without its mention being exclusively related to cancer), you'll notice a few strange things about the way authors deal with the subject. Many impart a homophobic tone that makes even *me* wonder if I'm repressing anything—and this goes for both male and female authors. It's as if they wanted you to be absolutely sure they're straight when they're telling you about what's inside guys' butts, and that you are too, and that every-one's still straight after they read about it.

The concept of male anal penetration obviously carries a lot of stigma and shame for these authors. This would be funny if it weren't so frustrating trying to get practical sex information out of their books. The other unfortunate thing most books do when they cover real-life, try-this-at-home prostate stimulation (which is rare) is rush through the material and present it in a cold context, as if no one would really try this for pleasure. Oh, and did I mention that prostate play, or the enjoyment thereof, has nothing to do with sexual orientation? It doesn't. End of discussion.

Myths about Getting Pegged

It's not just the authors of sex guides who worry about what it might mean when a straight guy likes anal play. Men often like to play with all parts of themselves when they masturbate, yet they might never confess a fantasy of sharing this pleasure in fear of partner judgment and/or coming to terms with social sexual stigmas. Women might be interested in trying it because they read or heard from a friend that it's like a secret pleasure weapon—but they may be worried about what it might mean for him, for them as a couple, and whether or not it's safe or clean to try. Mostly, it all boils down to fear of the unknown and believing the hype about male sexuality and anal play. Let's look at the myths surrounding strap-on play for couples.

> Prostate play has nothing to do with sexual orientation.

It means he's actually gay.

When a man wants a woman to strap on a synthetic penis and penetrate his anus, it means he wants a woman to fuck him up the ass. If he wanted a man to do it, he could find another man to do so with relative ease. Pegging isn't a "gateway" for homo-sexuality: gay men fantasize about, have sex with and fall in love with other men. They don't ask women to buy sex toys and have sex with them. A desire for anal sex has nothing to do with sexual orientation.

He can't be satisfied with "normal" sex.
Actually, it's a sex act couples add when they're totally satis-fied with their sexual routines—it doesn't diminish the value of your other sexual variations or mean that anyone's unhappy with the way things are going. Since all variations of sex out-side of heterosexual missionary intercourse fall outside the "normal" category, this could just as easily be said of oral sex—like all sexual variations couples share, strap-on sex is just another variation in the contemporary definition of "normal" sex. Sex is a buffet of many different pleasures, and this is just another side dish couples enjoy once in a while (or a lot if they think it's yummy). When you try pegging and find you like it, you may find yourselves doing it with frequency, until it becomes part of your routine sexual choices.

Once you try it, you'll only want more extreme things.
That's like saying people who like hot sauces will only be happy when they set their tongues on fire with gasoline and a road flare. Discovering that you enjoy strap-on play doesn't give you the unquenchable desire to try things that are crazier, harder, extreme, dangerous or addictive—but if you grow comfortable with it, you will crave variation, like trying different dildos, or new fantasies. Urges for extreme sex play already exist before someone buys a sex toy or she sticks a dildo in his butt for fun.

Anal sex is painful.

When it's done properly, anal penetration doesn't hurt *and* it feels incredibly good. Many people try anal sex without understanding that it requires lots of lube and patience (slowness), and that the recipient absolutely must be sexually aroused to even begin—and he or she has to really want to be doing it in the first place. Anal sex hurts when you go too fast, you need more lube, someone's not ready yet, or he really doesn't want to be doing it at that moment. It feels very intense for the first few minutes of penetration because of all the nerve endings concentrated in the anus—but in an instant, it feels *intensely good*.

It'll stretch out the anus.

This is a very hurtful myth, right up there with the myth of vaginas getting all stretched out from "too much" sex or promiscuity. Like the vagina, the rectum is amazing in its capacity to relax; stretch its muscles, ligaments and skin; and then retract back to its regular state. Its *function* is to do this. During arousal and anal penetration, everything expands to accommodate whatever is providing the pleasurable stimulation—nothing is being torn, stretched, or permanently worn out. In fact, regular stimulation of blood flow through arousal and penetration serves to make the area and organs surrounding it healthier, the muscles stronger and more resilient.

It's dirty and disgusting.

Other than the lube you'll get everywhere, anal sex is a pretty clean activity if you prepare for it. Concerns about anal cleanliness can be alleviated in a variety of ways. Taking a shower or bath and washing the anus thoroughly will make the outer rectum squeaky clean—and you can even start your anal play in the shower if you're interested in a totally clean experience. Using gloves for finger play and condoms on sex toys can make cleanup a snap, and you can always put a towel down if you're worried about sleeping in lube. Having your lover use the restroom to be sure he's "all clear" for a strap-on landing is a prerequisite, and will ensure that your experience will be typically mess-free. An enema is one option for absolute surety, but it's never really necessary. Either way, you're going to get messy with lube that has anal bacteria in it

> When it's done properly, anal penetration doesn't hurt *and* it feels incredibly good.

(even if everything looks totally clean), so do make sure your toys get cleaned thoroughly afterward, and don't touch the vaginal area with anything that came in contact with the butt. However, if you just plain think that the ass is a disgusting thing—don't look behind you.

Chapter 3

Male Pleasure Anatomy

It's no myth that anal sex feels good, yet for men there is much more to the anal pleasure inventory than for us gals: thanks to the prostate gland, when a man reaches the summit of pleasure through anal stimulation, he gets a lot more than a great view. Orgasmically speaking, when a man comes from anal stimulation, he gets the most explosively exuberant sunrise—an unbelievably deep and powerful orgasm, every time he makes the well-lubed trek.

The Prostate

The prostate gland is the celebrity star of the male body. It is at once supervillain and action hero: the site of a common threat of cancer, and the possible promise of legendary pleasures. Rebuked, reviled, redeemed, and romanced, this little gland manages to make headlines when viewed from any angle. Sometimes the attention is conflicted: the gland makes prostatic fluid for carrying virile semen, making the man "a man";

it also makes orgasm outrageously powerful but requires access through anal penetration, questioning some people's definition of "a man." The world of medicine would have us think of the prostate in only the most functional terms: in connection with embarrassing health treatments; as a primordial DNA delivery service.

But in fact the prostate is a symphony of packaging, form and function. Design Within Reach has nothing on this Deco-reminiscent heart-shaped secretory gland—*gland*, as in glandular—*secretory*, literally "relating to or promoting secre-tion." In its jaunty seat within the command center of the male pleasure system, the prostate gland is located inside the per-ineal wall, nestled within the internal root of the penis. It sits just below the bladder, producing the fluid that mixes with semen in ejaculate (and that lusciously lusty liquid evidence of male arousal, pre-come), and is connected to the urethra, the muscles that line the perineum, and the sphincter muscle.

If there's an epicenter to male orgasm, then the prostate must be it. Many men, though not all, find that when they're aroused, prostate stimulation is intensely pleasurable; that's because the nerve pathway from the brain to the penis runs through the rectum, and one large nerve bundle is located just beneath the prostate. Because the penis is more or less anchored at the prostate, when you massage the prostate you also trans-mit sensation to the base of his penis. So, to truly understand why a finger in the ass during a blowjob might work like a magic button to make him come, or why he leaves his body during orgasm when you fuck him with that turquoise dildo, let's look at the entire male pleasure system, and the prostate's smug little role in all of it.

His External Pleasure Anatomy: Penis and Testicles

Contrary to marketing stereotypes, men cannot be stimulated to orgasm with horsepower, touchdowns or swimsuit editions— the wick of Eros may be lit above the shoulders, but it glows at crotch level, thank you very much. You might think that it's a simple affair; that like all of its correspondingly yawn-worthy phallic allegories of guns and hoses, getting a guy off is as simple as "unzip fly, aim, and shoot." But as we'll see, a cigar isn't always a cigar, and not only is the male pleasure system deliciously con-nected and complex, but the packaging is exciting, versatile, and rejoices in delightful deviance.

Men's genitals all begin from the same stuff in utero (à la the fetal gen-ital ridge), but as a boy grows into the uniqueness that is him, his parts grow with him and become as unique to him

> The prostate is the epicenter of male orgasm.

as his face and fingerprints. Though there are infinite variations, what you will generally encounter when you slide the man out of his Calvins is: a penis (circumcised or not), a scrotal sack containing two testicles, and pubic hair that usually covers the mound over the pubic bone, the base of the penis, the testicles, and the perineum (from the base of the balls to the anus). The skin on the pubic mound, the perineum, and the anus is simi-lar in texture to the skin on the rest of his body, but usually a different shade. It deepens and changes in color as it reaches the base of the penis and the scrotum. The darker skin is softer and thinner than the skin on the rest of his body.

There are many nice things about penises—especially the fact that each man has his very own. Penises come in a variety of shapes and sizes. The range of sensation, size and responsiveness is also different for each man and depends on various factors—so rule number one is that you can't predict anything based on the way a penis looks. They also vary greatly in size, both in flaccid (soft) and erect (hard) states. The size of a man's soft penis is not a reliable gauge of its erect state, or attitude once fully hard; it could have the body of a supermodel but the brain of a...supermodel. It could be Clark Kent, Dr. Jekyll, Diana Prince...

Penises come in more shapes, sizes and variations than words can communicate—though there certainly has been a lot written about them.

Powers of transformation aside, the base of the penis sprouts from the pubic mound, which is usually covered with hair—it can be thick as a forest, or thin and barely there; and how he styles it can vary from *au naturel* to trimmed, shaved or even waxed. The skin covering the pubic bone (or pubic mound) is generally fleshier than any of the skin surrounding it, and the mound is where the skin begins to deepen in color as it meets the base of the penis. The shaft of the penis begins just below the pubic bone and continues internally almost all the way to the anus. This part of the penis can't be sized up through jeans, or compared in the locker room; rather than a private joke, it's more like a secret smile.

Penises come in more shapes, sizes and variations than words can communicate—though there certainly has been a lot written about them. The skin covering a man's penis is almost always darker in tone than the skin everywhere else (though sometimes it's lighter), and it's smoother in texture. Colors can range from the lightest pink to the deepest chocolate and anywhere in between. The color at the tip, also called the *head*, or *glans*, will generally differ from the rest of the penis, especially his circumcision scar if he has one, and penises are seldom the same color all over. Shapes are yet another variable: he can be thick at the base and slender at the tip, wide from top to bottom; have a wide head but a shaft that is slender in girth, or any number of other combinations, each of which is perfectly normal. The color, size and shape of a man's penis has nothing to do with how he responds to your stimulation—or what type of lover he is.

Hot dog, cannon, skyscraper, or train; tasty, scary, swaggering, stereotypical—a phallus is still just a phallus. The penis is essentially a long shaft, or tube, that ends at the tip with the urethral opening, where urine and ejaculate (sperm or "come") leave the body. Inside the penis, the urethra continues as a long tube through the center of two other larger tubes of spongy erectile tissue, whose proper names are *corpus cavernosum* and *corpus spongiosum*. When arousal triggers an erection, these tissues fill with blood, hardening the shaft and head of his penis. However, an erection does not always indicate whether a man is aroused; he can be perfectly, happily aroused and remain unerect.

Tasty, scary, swaggering, stereotypical— a phallus is still just a phallus.

At the tip is where you'll find the head, or glans. The head has the largest concentration of nerve endings in the penis, and it can be very responsive to stimulation—and sometimes extremely sensitive to touch (especially after orgasm). Always ask your partner what level of stimulation of the head of his cock works for him at any given time, because his preference levels will change throughout the pleasure cycle. The head is often bulbous—anywhere from slightly to quite pronounced. If he's uncircumcised, in its soft state the head will be covered in a thin jacket of skin called a *foreskin*. As his penis becomes aroused, the glans will harden and emerge. In North America, most infant boys are circumcised, a process in which the foreskin is removed shortly after the bundle of joy first sees the light of his new world—and perhaps regrets not getting a round-trip ticket.

Beneath the head of his cock is usually the most sensitive part, which some men claim is their "sweet spot," the spot they really enjoy having touched when they're aroused. This spot can range in location from just at the urethral opening to farther down the underside of the shaft, where circumcised men will have a bas-relief scar in memory of the foreskin. On an uncircumcised man, this spot runs along the same area, beneath the tip of the cockhead, from the urethral opening (underside) to approximately where the inner skin of the foreskin's hood becomes the outer skin of the penis.

Underneath the penis is where we find the scrotal sack, containing the two testicles—or not. Not all men have a pair, and some inherit a trifecta of fruit and get three for the price of admission. Men can indeed have one, two, or more testicles from the time they are born, or they might later have one (or more) removed for medical reasons, such as cancer. These are the "balls." Their wrinkly, fleshy container, the *scrotum* (or scrotal sack), hangs attached at the base of his penis and can be the same color as the penis or darker in tone. With rare exceptions, the testicles are usually covered with a lighter covering of hair than the pubic bone, yet they can sometimes be just as furry. Most men's testicles hang unevenly; one is usually lower than the other.

To "testify" is to swear upon the truth of your words; the word comes from the male ritual of gripping their most prized possession while making an oath, or swearing upon their sexual chestnuts, as it were. I swear on my nutsack to tell the truth, the whole truth. Of course, we're talking about the scrotum, which is the container of loose, thin skin that holds the testicles inside. Its unusual characteristic is the *cremaster muscle*, which causes the testicles to wrinkle here and there and to go up and down as they contract and relax. It's really a heat regulator: when it's chilly, the muscle will pull the scrotum up and bring the testicles closer to the body, and when the temperature rises, it relaxes and lets them hang. When he's about to ejaculate, the muscle retracts, pulling the testicles close to the base of the penis, as if to say, *I swear this is going to feel really good.*

It may seem like all they do is hang around waiting for something to happen, but the testicles are like a continually running software program, quietly performing many functions in the background while we're all online browsing cock. These small, egg-shaped spheres feel uneven and bumpy in texture when you touch them through the skin, but that's because they're tightly wound masses that consist of tubes—similar to a rubber-band ball. Between the tubes are cells that produce that celebrity hormone testosterone, and the tubes themselves are where sperm are born and bred. The sperm travel from the tubes through a lumpy mass at the back of the testicle that's actually one long coiled-up tube, and into the fast freeway of the *vas deferens.* Destination: urethra.

A man's testicles are very sensitive to the touch, but many men enjoy having them caressed, lightly massaged, or even gently tugged or pulled during foreplay and arousal. Most men will not enjoy having them slapped, spanked or roughly pulled— but there are exceptions, and this type of pleasure play should be expressly discussed in advance. Generally, you should treat them like a pair of delicate eggs.

Behind the testicles and between the thighs is a flat stretch of skin that's also covered with hair and often the same color as the penis—this is his *perineum*. Beneath the skin of the perineum is where the root, or bulb, of the penis lies, and when he gets an erection you can feel this area harden too. Stroke or rub this area during other sexual stimulation, and you will probably get a positive response—in part, because you are indirectly massaging his prostate.

Chapter 4

The Anus and Prostate

S urprisingly little is known about the prostate gland's pleasure purposes. It produces prostatic fluid (which comprises
up to a third of the liquid volume in ejaculate), it grows as a
man ages (sometimes dangerously), and in case you missed every
page of this book so far—it can feel really, really good when
sexually stimulated. It's clear that it plays an important role in
the male pleasure cycle, and it has become touted as the male
G-spot. Some call it the "P-spot." When a man reaches the point
of orgasmic "no return" (ejaculatory inevitability), the prostate
gland joins the seminal vesicles and other ducts in a little do-
si-do of pleasant-feeling spasms and rhythmic contractions to
create ejaculate—and this is before the contractions of orgasm.
If you are stimulating a man's prostate prior to and during ejaculation, you can often feel the gland swell to hardness, then
contract before his orgasm.

The Male G-Spot

The prostate gland is within the front wall of the anal opening, usually around one to three inches inside and forward (toward the front of the body or belly button). Its location inside the wall is just behind the bulb of the penis, beneath the bladder, surrounding the urethra in a ring. Because the prostate is anchored at the internal base of the penis, when a man thrusts hard with an erect penis he transmits highly pleasurable sensations to the prostate. It's a little larger than a quarter in size, though it is heartshaped and usually described as being the size of a small walnut.

One of the reasons that a man might like anal play is that massaging the prostate gland feels incredibly pleasurable and can make orgasm very powerful. But he might also like it because the anus and anal opening are rich with nerve endings that feel good to the touch; the 15,000 pudendal nerve fibers that wire and electrify the entire pelvis interact with the nerve bundles in the anus and prostate. There are also psychological factors in play here—what's a filthier insult than ass, what's dirtier than shit, what's as insultingly feminine as penetration (and liking it)? He may like that it's a big taboo, that it's a "dirty" thing to do; maybe no one touches him there and it means a lot to have you care about his pleasure; or it may be part of a Dominant/submissive fantasy scenario in which he "makes" you do it, or you "make" him submit to it. One thing is certain—the men who like anal stimulation like it a lot, and for many of these men, prostate stimulation can turn an orgasm into an unforgettable experience.

> Men like anal play because massaging the prostate gland feels incredibly pleasurable.

But wait—ass class is still in session: the perineum stretches from the base of the testicles to the anus, where it is no longer perineum and definitely ass. It has some hair, either a light, downy covering, or a thick, coarse carpet—it's different on every man. Between his cheeks, you'll see the anal opening, a pucker that will differ in color from the skin on the rest of the body. In fact, it's common for the thin skin surrounding the pucker to be lighter or darker in color between the cheeks.

Like the prostate, penis and most internal organs of the body, the anus is controlled by what are known as "smooth muscles," meaning that they're not striated nor are they bulkable like biceps, and like any smooth or shifty character, they are indeed out of your control. So flexing a cock won't make it bigger, and having anal orgasms won't give you "six-pack" butt muscles—though an increase in orgasmic muscle tone is good for all pelvic functions and healthy for stimulating blood flow to the genital region. Interestingly, there are several sphincter muscles in the human body (like the iris of the eye), but the ones that matter here are the two anal sphincter muscles, the inner, which is smooth and involuntary, and the outer, which is under voluntary control and will more or less behave when you tell it to.

> One thing is certain—the men who like anal stimulation like it a lot.

The anal opening is packed with nerve endings that make it pleasurable to play with when the owner is aroused. Anal play is fun and feels good if you play according to the terrain; the anus is not self-lubricating so you must always use lots of lube. The skin is thin and tears easily so you have to touch and penetrate with items that are absolutely smooth. The muscles are sometimes slow to relax, so you too must be slow to invade their space. And because the inner muscles are involuntary, they push and pull things in and out as they please, so you must take care never to insert items that could get "lost" in the rectum. Because then, you and your smooth operators will wind up in the ER. Read all about anal sex safety and guidelines for hot penetration in chapter 8.

How to Find the Prostate with Your Eyes Closed

While this all may seem like a guide to safer spelunking rather than down and dirty fucking alfresco, you really don't need a flashlight to find the prostate, or to be a sex expert to make it feel wonderful as you go along in search of the prize. To feel the prostate, insert a well-lubricated finger inside his anal opening and stroke toward the front of his body, in a "come-hither" motion. It may be too soft to feel easily in its unaroused state; in fact, you may not be able to feel it at all until he becomes aroused, when it swells and hardens. Similarly to the G-spot in women, stroking the prostate may trigger the feeling of needing to urinate. For men who aren't ready for penetration, you can stimulate the prostate indirectly by massaging the perineum in firm circles with the flat of your thumb. Some men like perineum massage only when they're aroused, and some don't like it at all—when in doubt, ask.

Beneath your fingers you'll feel that the gland is rounded, shaped like a walnut, but slightly cleaved down the center so it has a furrowed seam and two subtle halves that can be felt with the pad of your finger (when touched from inside the anus).

When he's aroused, it swells and becomes firm to the touch, and it's a lot easier to feel it. Plus, it's much more fun to touch when he's hot and bothered.

Apart from possibly making him feel like peeing, touching his prostate will certainly make him experience a fullness and pressure that he can feel in his penis. Juicy men who are prone to leaking pre-come may leak a little more when you massage their prostate; that's because the prostate is where the fluid comes from. Massage it gently but firmly; you can simply move your finger in the come-hither motion, or you can keep your curved finger stiff and move it in and out. As he gets close to orgasm the gland will swell more, and it will get quite hard before he ejaculates. Summit, reached; view, breathtaking.

Chapter 5

How Pegging Works (Oh So Well)

If the ultimate purpose for the prostate feeling so insanely good to stimulate remains a mystery, we can at least smile quietly to ourselves while we revel in such mysteries of the unknown—as long as we can exploit its pleasures with strap-ons, fingers, butt plugs and more. Because we don't need to know the cosmic "why" to get the ultimately rewarding "how"—and of course, the orgasmically explosive "how-to." Unsolved mysteries aside, let's mine this thing for all it's worth; damn the silicone torpedoes, full speed ahead.

So Much More than a Hard-on: Understanding the Arousal of Strap-On Sex

There is no single, general answer as to why it turns some men on to think about being fucked up the ass by their female lovers, and gets them off big-time to do it, because each man's sexual arousal factors are unique. It's not as obvious as jacking off to a naked girl, nor can it be understood entirely by exploring anal eroticism—some men who like strap-on sex don't fancy the idea of playing with the exit hatch, but relish the thought of high heels on a girl wearing a big fake black cock.

As good as anal sex feels, and with the added bonus of the prostate sweetening the deal, the lure of pegging is often more mental and emotional than physiological. Of course, once it's been tried with success, the pure pleasure from the sex act might become one of the main reasons for repeat play. But pegging both delivers anal pleasure and plays on a key component of pivotal arousal experiences: fantasy. And understanding male arousal is how you can make his pegging experiences unforgettable.

Male arousal is a complete bodily takeover, though the head and heart are often essential players in the arousal symphony. When a man becomes aroused, his senses magnify; his sense of smell is heightened, colors are brighter, his skin becomes more sensitive and responds readily to touch. If a hot chick in a strap-on was sexy to him before he got turned on, she's a thousand times sexier once his cock is hard, and his focus is hormonally sharpened on just one thing: her, and the urgent need to get a taste of her cock. Meanwhile, his internal and external sexual anatomy is responding—big-time. Many different muscles involuntarily tense, resulting in contractions of facial and abdominal muscles. His breathing becomes heavier, his core body temperature rises, his heart rate increases, his nipples may become erect, and some men get a sex flush across their chest, neck, face, and stomach. And if his cock hardens, the head darkens in color and his testicles swell and move close to his body.

Strap-On Sex and Erection

It's not just that his cock gets hard and he wants to try something kinky—not at all. Physical arousal comes from two sources in varying measures and combinations, each a requirement for the other—mentally, from his brain, or physically, from his body's response to stimulation. In any given instance, fantasy may be fueling the fires more than touch, or vice versa. His mind and body work in tandem to make him hot under the collar and hard under the Calvins—you can have one without the other and still be aroused, but then, well, you have one and not the other. These two factors (in whatever proportion) trigger neural responses along nerve pathways that widen the arteries leading to the penis and other erectile tissue. Blood begins to flow into his penis and its underground erectile tissue, and his penis and perineum begin to harden. The prostate starts to grow firm to the touch.

Blood flows into the main tubes of the penis, creating rigidity as the flow of blood expands the erectile tissue, trapping the blood in his penis, creating and sustaining the erection until the nerve messages stop, or he ejaculates. (The nerve pathways for erection and ejaculation are different, which is why a man can ejaculate without erection and vice versa.) The blood flowing to his genitals is also being trapped inside the bulb and root of his penis, contributing to a firmer perineum.

To make an erection, the blood swells the tissue inside until it strains against the sheath of skin covering the penis. Lo, it is risen. What's important to remember when you're pegging, is that he won't always have a hard cock when you're fucking him. He might start out with a softie and get hard later, or he might lose his erection, yet confusingly tell you he's loving it and don't stop, please, no really. That's because as his pleasure cycle moves up and down the peaks and valleys of arousal, so will his erection grow soft and firm again. In prolonged sexual encounters like strap-on sex, it's not uncommon for erections to come and go as the pegging progresses, and this normal cycling has nothing to do with his actual arousal or desire.

When you're pegging him and he gets close to orgasm, you'll observe a number of physical signs, though they may not be all the ones you're used to seeing during your typical lovemaking rituals. Muscle tension builds to a pinnacle as he reaches the point of no return. His glans is very sensitive to stimulation, and both penis and shaft become very hard, as does the prostate. The testicles pull up very close to his body, contributing a delicious pressure. His breathing is labored, his blood pressure is up, and the skin all over his body is electric and extremely sensitive. His whole body is flooded with potent sexual chemicals, coloring his vision with nothing but the demands of getting more of whatever is pushing him onward; this often results in him backing up against your strap-on, thrusting wildly (making it hard to ride 'em, cowgirl), or physically flattening out in a facedown position. He might moan loudly or not at all; he might ejaculate wildly or in a way barely noticeable. Most often, there is much yelling and remarkable squirting, unless he's already come once before your cock and his ass have made their introductions.

The Mechanics of Orgasm

Inside, a different orgasmic story is told. As his arousal heightens, all the muscles and ligaments in the genital region begin to tighten, creating an exquisite tension—tension that sings to the tune of the fullness and rhythm created by strap-on penetration. The prostate gland is swollen with fluid, waiting for the signal to begin its orgasmic contractions; at this time of pressure and firmness, the internal massage from a well-wielded dildo feels incredible. As he gets closer to orgasm the figure eight of muscles that surround the penile system and ring the anus become tense, constricting and wringing more pleasure from the dildo (or plug, or fingers) and making his entire lower body part of the pleasure process. Before the peak, the prostate gland shudders and releases the prostatic fluid to mix with semen and other juices—this is "orgasmic inevitability," the point when a man knows he is about to come, and nothing on earth can stop it. During the orgasmic phase of sexual response, when a man feels orgasmic inevitability, the fluids that comprise ejaculatory fluid are being pushed into the prostatic urethra. Then the short, rhythmic muscular contractions of orgasm begin, not just in the penis but also throughout the entire genital region (including both sphincter muscles), and he orgasms, usually with ejaculation. Some men will want you to keep thrusting during orgasm to complete the sensations, and for these guys it makes the orgasm even more intense to feel thrusts during contractions. Others might want you to hold still, or move more slowly—pay close attention when he comes and continue the motions you made when he started coming until you "tune in" to what he likes best. Better yet, ask him what he might like, even when he's coming. He may want something different each time; asking him lets him control the sensation, proceeding on your own keeps you in control—it's a variable for you both to play with.

Men who ejaculate expel different amounts, but it's usually around one to two teaspoons. The volume can change depending on frequency (whether he's come recently, or not in a long time), stress, or other factors. Come is comprised of plasma, fluid from the prostate and seminal vesicles, around ninety million sperm, and other fluids that contain fructose, protein, citric acid, alkalines, and other nutrients that keep sperm intact. It can also contain HIV and sexually transmitted diseases, if he's infected. Come is usually whitish in color, but the color can also be varying degrees of clear, white, or yellow. The texture is that of a slightly thick liquid substance, somewhere between egg whites and hair conditioner, though some men might have very thick come while others' is thin. The muscular force with which his come is shot makes the difference in distance (if you're measuring), and some guys shoot pretty far, while with others our phallic metaphors stay holstered, as it were, and there is no shooting going on at all.

> "Orgasmic inevitability" is the point when a man knows he is about to come, and nothing on earth can stop it.

Fantasies and Realities of Pegging

As I mentioned earlier in this chapter, fantasy plays a huge role in strap-on sex—for his arousal, and yours as well. He might fantasize about the powerful woman who dominates him and takes what she wants, owning every inch of him, as it were, making him into her total submissive plaything. Or he might get excited about having something "dirty" done to him, beyond or within his control. It might just be the all-out kinkiness of seeing his hottest girl sporting the contrast of a phallus—with intent. His fantasy might hinge around anal sex against his will. All based around an enjoyment of anal stimulation, he could frame the encounter as a doctor or nurse exam, a prison encounter, a punishment, or a reward. It could also be sweet and loving, two people sharing the intimacy of penetration.

Similarly for the woman wielding the dick: the reverse of all these fantasies could be true and more. But unlike the recipient of the pegging, she needs to be the one controlling not just the rubber dick between her legs, but the realistic parameters of getting that thing in him safely and pleasurably, and ensuring that a good time is had by all.

> Discussing anal play before you try it is advised, unless you and your lover already have sexual adventure and exploration on the table.

Of course, that means no surprises when it comes to strap-on sex. Discussing anal play before you try it is advised, unless you and your lover already have sexual adventure and exploration on the table. Anal play for someone who's not ready for it can be very unsettling; don't just guess how he might react, because for some guys, anal penetration is going too far.

In reality there are three general rules for anal penetration: go very slowly, listen to the person you're penetrating, and use lots of lube. Sex toys used for anal penetration must have a flared base, meaning a base that prevents them from being pulled into the anal canal, where they can get lost—a nightmare waiting to happen. The sphincter muscles have minds of their own and like to squeeze and contract at will; we cannot control them. This serves to push and pull things in and out of the anus, and once something gets pulled in, there's no guarantee you're going to get it out without a trip to the hospital—which is what you'd have to do to prevent serous injury if, say, a hot, battery-powered vibrator went AWOL. Take a look at a standard butt plug and you'll see exactly what a flared base should look like.

Another reality to add to your fantasies: always use lots of lubrication—the skin around the anus tears easily, but won't if it's lubed enough. Also, never put something in someone's butt that has sharp edges; can possibly break, shatter or crack; or doesn't have a significantly flared base for easy retrieval. A tiny cut inside the rectum can easily become infected with fecal matter and can lead to more serious infections involving other organs in the body, which could lead to life-threatening situations if left untreated. Of course, caution and health concerns won't be the only reason you use lube, and lots of it—the slick, delicious sensation of erotic massage (with a dildo, natch) when everything is slippery is mind-blowingly arousing. Lube transmits and increases pleasurable touch like nothing else, and once you try it, you'll watch your lube bills go up with quite a contented smile on your face. There is nothing like sex with slicked-up parts, period.

Sex on Wheels

Alison Tyler

WHEN MILA ANNOUNCED that she wanted to spend the day cleaning the garage, I groaned. Here was something I seriously was not looking forward to. Who wants to waste a perfectly good weekend day doing a chore that has *drudgery* written all over it? Aside from that, our garage is a nightmare, filled with our favorite outdoor toys, all jumbled together in a giant mess. But something about the smirk on her pretty face let me know that I should go along with her desires, that I shouldn't bother listing all of the things I'd rather do.

Once in the garage, I waited for her to give me an assignment. When she didn't, I simply began puttering over in one corner, halfheartedly rearranging our climbing cables and harnesses, trying to find places for our various sporting equipment. We're both outdoorsy, and we really need a whole room for all of our various athletic gear, but we just don't have the space.

After a few minutes, Mila said, "Alan, will you do me a favor?"

I looked over at her questioningly.

"Slip on your Rollerblades." She had them in her hands. "Why?"

"Just do it."

I shrugged, kicked off my sneakers and laced on the skates. In a flash, Mila was at my side, pulling my cargos down my thighs, bending me over the hood of our car and rocking her sweet supple body against me.

Immediately, I realized that she was packing.

"Jesus," I sighed, "what's up with you?" I didn't mind. Of course, I didn't. But she'd caught me by surprise.

"I had this fantasy," she said, pressing her cock against me. "Of fucking you on wheels."

My heart started racing. I couldn't believe that I'd missed the signs. When Mila had suggested we spend the day cleaning, I'd instantly gotten lost in a gray haze. But now I realized that my sultry wife had given me clues as to her real motives. She wasn't dressed for cleaning, first of all. She had on a sexy lavender skirt, a tight-fitting tank top, and tie-up sandals. There was nothing about her attire or her attitude that should have led me to believe we'd be spending the day scrubbing.

"You look so fucking sexy in those," she said, her mouth pressed up against my ear. "I'm always wanting to fuck you when you have them on."

She bent down then, and reached for something I couldn't see. But I could guess what she was after. Lube. Within a few seconds, I knew I was right. The cold smear of the thick liquid around my naked asshole made me tremble. Tremble, and then tighten up.

"Relax, baby," Mila crooned. "It's always so much easier when you let yourself go. When you let me do what I want to do."

She was right, and I did my best. But still, when Mila slid two of her long, slim fingers inside of me, I clamped down hard.

"Come on, Alan. You know how much you want this."

She spoke the truth. I love when my girl takes charge. There is nothing sexier to me than when she shows up in our bedroom doorway, dressed for sex in a harness and one of her sturdy cocks. Yet it never gets easier for me to open up and take it. Mila always needs to soothe away my fears, to coax me over that first, difficult step.

Slowly, I let her fingers in deeper; slowly, I felt myself getting ready for the next stage of the game. Mila pressed me hard against the roof of our car. I could feel her cock gently probing forward, and then—with one thrust—she was in.

"Oh, fucking god," I groaned, demolished by the sensation. "You like that?"

I couldn't lie to her. "Yes."

She slid in deeper, and I groaned even harder. At first, she went easy on me. Mila knows how to open me up, to relax me with the tender way she works her toy inside of me. But when I began to beat my hips against the metal hood of the car, unable to stop myself, she started to speed up the rhythm. She could tell I was ready to handle a different sort of beat. With each thrust, she pulled me back against her, using the wheels on my skates to propel me. It felt wild, being a wheeled creature at the whim of her direction.

Was this what she had fantasized about? Why had she never said so before? We're a very open, playful couple. I would have happily allowed her to live out her fantasy. But maybe there was more. Or maybe the surprise aspect was part of the thrill for her.

I had let myself relax into the sensation for several seconds when suddenly, she pulled out.

"No," I moaned. "Don't stop."

"Shh," she chided me. "I have other plans." Slowly, she guided me, in a graceful slide, over to my workbench.

Now, she looped a length of climbing cable around my wrists and then tossed it over the rafter, pulling it back down and anchoring me. With the skates still on my feet, and my wrists over my head, I was actually pretty stable if totally in her power.

"Christ, you're pretty," she grinned, looking up at me. "Maybe I'll leave you like that."

"Don't you dare."

Mila dropped to her knees on the grease-stained concrete and started to blow me. I was dripping pre-come with excitement, a near wreck from the pleasure she was giving me with her mouth and the thrill she'd already given me with her synthetic toy, which still bobbed between her thighs.

My whole world was focused on the warmth of her mouth around me, on the way her lips moved up and down my shaft. I groaned out loud when she used one hand to cup my balls, and my voice went hoarse when she dragged her short nails along that most tender skin.

"Now," she said, gazing up at me with her warm brown eyes. "Tell me what you want."

"What do you mean?" I was breathless, near begging. What did I want? I wanted to come.

"Do you want me to suck you off? Or do you want me to fuck you until you shoot your load?"

Oh, man. Hearing my sweet wife say those dirty words nearly did me in. But I knew what she wanted to hear—and I knew it was the same thing I wanted to say.

"Fuck me," I whispered.

"That's my boy," Mila grinned, standing once more and coming to take her place behind me.

I swallowed hard as she pressed the head of that toy against my back door. And then I bit down on a growl as she slid swiftly inside of me. There was no going slow now. There was just Mila, gripping my hips, pulling me on those skates in the exact rhythm that she craved. She was fucking me hard, yet using the motion of the wheels to help her get just the right beat. I had no say in the matter, my wrists high over my head, my body at her total whim.

And I loved every damn second of it.

"You gave me some grief," Mila whispered, "when I told you what I wanted."

I was confused for a moment. Then I realized she was talking about my reaction to cleaning out the garage.

"You didn't say exactly what the plans were," I reminded her.

"But you ought to trust me by now."

Mila had me there. I should have known that she'd never waste a day like this on the drudgery of cleaning. She's not any more domestic than I am. But suddenly I couldn't talk anymore. I was filled, captive, and on wheels. Each thrust sent all sorts of messages to my body, none of which was louder than this: I AM GOING TO COME!

I said the words to Mila, and she laughed, low and dark. "That's right, baby. Come for me."

It was heaven. Pure heaven. A strange exotic mixture of power, trust and unexpected pleasure. I came all over the workbench and the concrete floor, and as soon as I climaxed, Mila followed. I could tell that she was coming by the way she slammed her body against mine, sealing herself to me, pressing her clit firmly to the base of the dildo and groaning.

Mila let the pleasure work through the two of us, the tremors finally subsiding before she pulled out, let me loose, set me free.

And now, whenever she suggests we clean the garage, or attic, or basement, I'm always ready and willing to say, "Yesssssss."

Chapter 6

How to Ask for It

For a kiss, most often a tilt of the head, a lowering of the eyes, and leaning forward—lipward—will do the trick. For oral sex, it's entirely possible to spontaneously initiate the entire exchange without a word being said, from the minute you head southward to the gratifying moments of completion, lips locked on the object of joy. And many an intercourse (penis to vagina) experience has occurred without a whisper, though likely moans and grunts of assent could be heard. But no act of male anal penetration—especially strap-on sex—could happen without someone asking for it, and someone else asking how it's to be done.

Basically, if someone's going to get "done" and get done right, you have to talk about it. Oftentimes, one of you has a fantasy—be it from a video, story, rumor, or trip to a sex toy store and a fervid imagination—about trying pegging. Maybe he's always wanted it, or he's tried it before and liked it. Perhaps she's loved sharing this with her other male partners, or has enjoyed strap-on sex with her girlfriends, or has always thought it would be hot to wear the dick for a change. No matter where you come from with pegging, you have to ask for it. And that can be as scary, exciting, fun, naughty or taboo as the act itself.

How to Bring It Up

The intimacy, sexual communication and sexual closeness that pegging both requires and provides is unrivaled by other sex acts—there is nothing to compare it to. When you're with a new lover, asking for strap-on sex might be easy—you've got nothing to lose, or perhaps the attraction was openly sexual and sex talk was up front to begin with. Or, when things are all shiny and new, it could be too scary to risk opening up with your less conventional sexual fantasies and desires, out of fear that you might scare a good thing away.

If someone's going to get "done" and get done right, you have to talk about it.

Established couples run into the same fears and risks when one person wants to try strap-on sex and he or she doesn't know if the other one will be into it or not. Of course, the surprise many couples have is discovering that you both want to try this unconventional new sex act—and most of the time, it turns out you're really well matched to go on these wacky and hot sexual adventures together. Imagine being scared to ask, and then getting your nerve up to ask, and having the reaction be, "Yes! I'll get the lube! Wait—do we need to go shopping?"

That's the ideal situation, though in reality it's not always the case—the reality will most often be a mixed reaction of excitement and confusion—your lover will always, always have lots of questions whenever you ask to try a new sex act, whether it's pegging or spanking. Just summoning the courage to ask is nerve-wracking: you might be worried that he'll judge you, or see your desire to try something new and kind of kinky as a surprise—maybe she'll wonder if you've been hiding things from her the whole time you've been together. You may worry he'll freak out completely, or worse, that it'll break—not make—your relationship. Asking for what you want is always, always scary. Honesty is a brave thing, indeed.

So, how do you ask to be fucked up the ass, or to gain an all-access pass to your boyfriend's posterior? Not everyone is going to feel vulnerable asking to try strap-on sex; some will be empowered, most will feel finally free to truly express themselves sexually and many others are just going to finally get to play the way they've been dreaming of for so long. Sharing this fantasy, the intimacy and all that goes with strap-on sex, can make your relationship strong, vibrant and alive.

Sharing this fantasy, the intimacy and all that goes with strap-on sex, can make your relationship strong, vibrant and alive.

But whatever your situation, telling him or her you want to try something new sexually can feel stressful—and if your fantasy makes *you* uncomfortable, this is an understatement. In fact, even thinking about talking about sex is stressful sometimes! If you've never brought up the subject of sex with your partner, even though you've been having it together for months or years, don't worry—it's not that unusual. If you have what you consider a routine style of sex, telling your partner that you want something to change is scary, and starting a conversation about your desire to sexually experiment can make you feel vulnerable. This is especially true with sexual fantasies that predate your relationship. Opening yourself up and asking for something you want sexually takes courage—but it also gives you an opportunity to learn more about what your lover likes and dislikes.

Once you get your courage up to ask, that doesn't always mean you'll be met with enthusiasm, or if you are, that your lover will be able to execute your desires in the ways you want. If this is the case for you, in later chapters you'll find specific sections and resources referring to specific books, videos and websites to direct your sweetie to so he or she can learn more about how to give you what you want—and vice versa. But opening up can be scary, and meeting with shock, surprise, or distaste is even scarier. Learning how to talk about each other's desires, and picking up tips for starting the conversation, are where you'll want to begin.

> Start by whispering naughty ideas or scenes to each other during sex.

What If You Don't Normally Talk about Sex?

If you are new to talking about sex, try these starting points:

- Watch a film that has explicitly sexual scenes in it that are a bit kinkier than the usual fare, such as *Y Tu Mama Tambien, Secretary, Last Tango in Paris, Belle de Jour,* or *Mr. and Mrs. Smith.* Afterward, discuss the film and what in particular about it excited you.

- Give your lover a book of erotica for couples that contains stories with pegging in them, such as *Sweet Life: Erotic Fantasies for Couples, Taboo: Forbidden Fantasies for Couples,* and *She's On Top: Erotic Stories of Female Dominance and Male Submission.* Try reading stories aloud to each other to spark fantasies and conversation afterward.
- Start by whispering naughty ideas or scenes to each other during sex.
- Confess a fantasy that you'd like to try that incorporates light male anal play, like a blowjob with benefits—this will likely ignite some very hot sex.
- Explain in an intimate, private setting that you'd like to talk openly about your fantasies together, and discuss ways in which you'd like to make them more realistic—maybe even make them into reality.
- Propose that you each make a list of the five sexual fantasies that you'd most like to try, and then swap lists and discuss.

In some cases, you both already have ideas about what fantasies you'd like to try together. People who are lucky enough to find lovers that they click with on other levels often find that they sexually click too. Others, with a little sexual sleuthing, find out that their lovers are equally curious about the possible aphrodisiac effects of fantasies on their shared sex life, and that they too look forward to trying something new that could really spice things up.

If you're the one bringing it up, reverse roles for a minute: if you don't normally talk about sex in your relationship and then suddenly one of you wants to, it might be upsetting—at first. Consider ways in which you can encourage your partner to hear you out, and ask him to suspend judgment until you can explain why this is important, and how much fun you think the two of you will both have—and how important her participation is to you.

Think about what your lover's fears and concerns might be before you even bring it up—and feel free to hand her or him the "myths" chapter of this book, or the sexual anatomy chapters that explain why anal play feels good and is safe, and even the preparation section in chapter 8 to put any cleanliness fears to rest. Don't let your lover feel intimidated by your desire to peg or be pegged: reassure him or her that you find them incredibly sexy, and that this wouldn't be happening unless you felt safe to tell them your deepest desires. Your lover needs to hear that he or she is the star of your show, in addition to the fact that you're ready to become closer than you've ever been before. Rehearse what you'd like to say in your mind before you actually have the conversation. Think through possible scenarios, and imagine how your listener might react, so that you will be prepared to flow with whichever route the discussion might take.

And If the Reaction Is Negative?

Plainly put, since he's the one who would be penetrated, if he says no, then it's not going to happen. In reality, one of you may ask sweetly to try pegging, with candles and flowers and kisses and eager ideas—but may be met with a flat-out refusal. Don't give up just yet, but also react with compassion and understanding, even if it's logically confusing to you. For many reasons, one of you may not want to try strap-on sex; your lover may want to make you happy but not understand what to do, or what it means to you. Understanding these concerns and hesitations can be helpful in having a constructive discussion about it, learning how to overcome fears that might hold one of you back, and resolving what to do when one person does feels okay about it while the other doesn't.

If pegging is something you've requested but your partner is reluctant, be aware of the pressure he may be feeling; explore his concerns in conversation, and hand him a chapter of this book to read when he needs concrete answers about anything pertaining to male anal penetration and strap-on sex. And understand that some people may never feel completely comfortable with anal sex or dildo play or even sex toys, for whatever reasons, and that he or she will need to experience their feelings at their own pace.

Perhaps you're the one freaking out about your lover asking to try strap-on play. Anxiety can be no laughing matter when you're wondering about the details—the nitty gritty—of what your lover wants, or what it might mean. Get to the bottom of your stress by finding out what's interfering with your understanding of your partner's desire to try this new pleasure. Are you unsure about the notion that your partner wants to play with the "back door," let alone put a scary dildo in it? Take my word on it—our collective discomfort with our genitals, and gender play, and anal play for that matter, is not limited by gender. Everyone worries about smell, appearance, comparisons, and performance. And always, in every sex act—intention and true motivations.

For some people the idea of messing with traditional gender roles is beyond what they can deal with. And for some men, ass play is threatening to all the things they believe make them men. Pegging is generally culturally misunderstood; it triggers things we may not even understand ourselves, and just having these feelings or desires can make us feel sexually isolated—and may make us feel like bad people for enjoying them. A reactive lover might try to make you feel bad for even suggesting it—again, patience and compassion are key, even if his or her reaction doesn't make sense to you at the time.

It might be that the fantasy context your lover suggested for strap-on play is beyond what you deem acceptable. We all know that fantasy is not reality. But when we masturbate and imagine troubling things, people, or situations, our human curiosity kicks in and we ask ourselves whether these things are what we really want. For some people this is a horrifying thought. It's important to keep in mind that fantasies don't necessarily bear any relationship to reality. The realm of fantasy is the sanctuary in your mind where you are free to enjoy things that you would never do in real life. And fantasy is not only where we can court the forbidden, it is also a powerful sex toy that can be used to arouse, heighten pleasure, and achieve climax.

Relationships and arousal from fantasy may come from two different places, yet they aren't mutually exclusive—they can work together perfectly once you understand what fantasies are, and how to use them. With some fantasies, we can't help but indulge in them, nor can many of us resist getting aroused by them. And because we want our relationships to include every little thing that gets us hard or wet, the lack of control over fantasy and arousal can make us feel out of control. It's as if what's safe is always at odds with what is sexy, but it doesn't have to be. Two mature adults exploring their fantasies together can make things that seem scary—yet confusingly hot at the same time— a beautiful, hot, fun and repeatable experience for both of you.

Found Art

Alison Tyler

I'M A MASSEUSE by training, but I know how to touch people by nature. I've always been good at finding and exorcising the knots that hide beneath the skin. In a crazy town like Los Angeles, I consider myself blessed to have a skill that brings in good money while reducing people's stress.

For several years, I worked at a high-end salon. Now, I free-lance, traveling door-to-door to my clients' homes, bringing my table and my bag of tricks with me. I'm strong for my size—you have to be in my work—and I have capable hands. Plus, I possess a calm personality that puts my clients instantly at ease. I don't know if it's because I'm attractive, or because I can make people laugh. Regardless, it's an added benefit.

Once you get on my table, your problems melt away.

Although massages can be sexual, I do not give sexual massages to my clients. I am strictly professional. At least, I *was* until last weekend. I had been booked to do two massages at a house in the Hollywood Hills. These clients are among my favorites, a husband and wife who have been married for ten years (an eon in L.A.). He's an artist; she's a director. They possess completely opposite personalities. Within three minutes of climbing on my table, he falls asleep. I could get away with reading a book for the duration, although I give him the full treatment in spite of his snores. Alice is the opposite, a bundle of hard knots and live energy, and she talks her way through the entire massage.

When I arrived this weekend, they presented me with a surprise, asking if I could fit in a third party, a houseguest who
was staying over for the weekend.

"Sure," I said. "No problem."

"Thanks, Gabrielle," Richard grinned. "You're a doll."

I worked on Alice first, then Richard, and then they went
out to lunch while I did the third, an artist friend of theirs who
was visiting from Santa Fe. He was exactly my type, tall and
lean, with chiseled features, blue eyes, and long dark hair. Added
to those specs, he had a perfect body, and it was a pleasure oiling
him up and rubbing him down. He didn't say anything to me
for the first forty-five minutes of the massage. That's fine with
me. If clients want to talk, I'm ready to listen. If they don't, I
get lost in my work.

I had finished up with his shoulders, then his neck, then his
scalp, when he said, "You're good, you know it?"

"Thanks."

"No, really, this is the best massage I've ever had."

I smiled and kept working, thinking, *My pleasure*, but not
saying the words aloud, of course. I wasn't about to jeopardize
my steady job with my top clients, not for a quick tryst with
their houseguest, regardless of how appealing he was. But when
he rolled onto his back again and asked if I would spend a little
more time on the tops of his shoulders, I started to doubt my
own strength.

The sheet I'd draped over him had a floral pattern in dark
magenta over a pale pink background. Usually, I use plain white
sheets, but I had been extremely busy during the week and
hadn't gotten to the laundry in time to do a fresh set. The pattern was gaudy, and even more flagrant was his delicious

hard-on, pushing up from the sheet and making the fabric stand like a circus tent over his groin.

I didn't say anything, but my eyes returned to the tent repeatedly as I ran my hands over his shoulders in soothing strokes. He was definitely well-hung, and I had to keep searching for nonsexual thoughts while I worked. Traffic. Grocery shopping. Rollerblading. Nothing worked. Every time my eyes met that pup tent, it was all I could do not to reach one hand under the sheet and stroke him there.

But I was a good girl. I loosened the few remaining kinks in his shoulders, then worked out the knots, and when I was finished, I could feel the difference. He'd started out tense, as if someone had poured wet concrete between the grooves of his joints. Now, when I ran my fingers along his muscles, there was a give to them.

He opened his stunning ocean blue eyes and stared up at me, smiling. I smiled down at him, then took a step back, turning to look out the window at the hills below. I wanted to give him time to stand and wrap the sheet, or the towel his hosts had left for him, around his flat waist. I wanted to give him the privacy to get into some clothes before I took my table down.

"They won't be back," he said, and I felt a jolt within myself, felt my body responding to what I sensed was an offer. "They went to review the dailies for Alice's latest movie. She wanted Richard's opinion. They said they'd call me to tell me where to meet them for dinner."

I turned and faced him. He was sitting up on my table staring at me, one dark eyebrow cocked in an obvious invitation.

"I should really—" I started, thinking, *I should really just get the fuck out of here before I do something extremely foolish.*

"You should really let me work *you* for a while," he said, standing now and sliding on his silky emerald green boxers while I watched. He was built so nicely, and he was slow to pull those silk boxers up and over his raging hard-on.

"Work?" I asked, feeling ill-prepared for what was happening, caught so far off my guard.

"Let me give you a rubdown, in return. I'm pretty good." He stretched out the sheet and motioned for me to climb onto my own table. I hesitated, but he insisted. "I promise they won't come back. Don't worry—" and the other promise, the one in his voice, the one of impending sexual pleasures, decided it for me. I'd been on a sexual hiatus for the past few months. This was exactly what I craved.

With my heart in my throat, I took off my clothes and climbed onto the table. He oiled up his hands and began to work, thrilling me with the strength of his strokes. Most people are afraid to work deep, but he wasn't. He really pounded into me, knowing, somehow, that I like to be touched rough.

"What kind of artist are you?" I asked softly as his large, firm hands ran all the way under the sheet, cresting over the cheeks of my ass.

"I use found art," he said.

My mind took off to fantasyland, while I imagined exactly what that phrase might mean. *Found Art.* I tried to picture this stranger in his studio, touching objects with the same power with which he was touching me. And after a few minutes, I was practically purring, truly relaxed.

That is, until he reached into my bag on the pretext of grabbing another bottle of oil, and came up with something completely unexpected: a harness and dildo tucked into an inner pocket of my massage bag. I'd forgotten about those toys, remnants of a failed relationship.

"Found art," he murmured, echoing himself. I didn't know what he was referring to, but as I glanced at the prize in his hands, my cheeks turned as hot pink as the vibrant flowers on the sheet.

"I—" I stammered, but I didn't have anything to say after that. I *what*? I like to fuck men? It's true, but usually not the first thing out of my mouth with a potential lover.

"You—" he said, grinning. "You'd look absolutely luscious with this on."

I locked eyes with him, then sat up on the table. He handed over the toys, watching with appreciation as I stood, buckled the harness into place, then snapped the dildo on at the front.

How had we gotten here so quickly?

I had no idea. When I'd left for the morning's job, sex was the furthest thing from my mind. But now...now, with this stunning new man bending willingly over my table, with a bottle of lube that had been tucked next to the harness in the pocket, with hours until dinner...I had a completely different view of how the afternoon was going to turn out.

I started slowly. I oiled up the toy with the lubricant in my bag, then lubed up one of the two places on his body my hands had not yet found. He groaned as my fingers slid inside of his asshole. Then his head went down, and he sucked in his breath as I introduced him to the first bulbous inch of the dildo.

"Jesus..."

I went slowly at the beginning, until he murmured, "You worked me hard with the massage."

"Yes..."

"*That's* how I like to be fucked."

Now, I was the one to swear softly under my breath, because I couldn't believe my luck. My heart beat fiercely in my chest as I began to work him rougher, to slide that cock deep into his luscious ass. To pound into him with the ferocious rhythm of the blood in my own veins.

He stared out the windows at the hills while I fucked him. He stared at the trees in bloom, at the pale blue sky, at the puffs of clouds whispering by. I listened to the sound of his sweet breathing as I thrust the cock deep into his asshole and fucked him hard and fast.

"Oh, god," he groaned as I continued to work my hands over him while I fucked him, digging into his arms, my teeth searching for purchase on the ridge of his neck, my cock pummeling its way to deliverance inside the dark world of his ass.

He might have been an artist, but I was the one to use his body as a canvas. He might have been the one who worked with "found" materials, but as I made him come, I felt as if I were the true artiste.

He has a found art exhibition coming up at one of the modern art museums downtown.

I wonder what other inspirations the two of us will find.

Chapter 7

Communication Tips for Her and Him

If you're a woman reading this and you're the sexual initiator here, keep in mind as you start to talk about strapping it on and giving it to him that he's going to be having a number of fears, concerns and questions swirling around in his head. Be prepared to talk about everything, and also be prepared to be the one to bring up every little issue—even if he doesn't. You'll need to not only start the conversation but bring up a list of points in case he's too nervous or embarrassed to express his concerns. You want to be sure that all ground is covered here—from fear of pain and anal stretching myths to demasculinization—so that ultimately he'll make a positive decision because he wants to and not simply to please you.

You Want to, But He's Worried: Talking Points

If you're keen on trying strap-on play and he's unsure about it, make sure you talk about:

- Why this is hot and a turn-on for you.
- How it makes him even sexier in your eyes.
- Why anal penetration isn't painful when it's done correctly.
- Why anal pleasure does not lead to a stretched-out butt (see chapter 2 for facts).
- How it can make him come really hard.
- Why it doesn't make him gay or bisexual, nor does it make him less of a man. He'll be the same straight guy as before, just with a hotter (and more sophisticated) sex life.
- Whether or not this will be a domination and submission scenario. Some men will like that aspect, some men will dislike the idea strongly.
- The fact that this is a very intimate act that you hope will bring you closer together.
- The way you don't find his genitals—especially his ass—gross or dirty, and that you're not squeamish about the details of anal play.

Let's flip this for a minute—let's say it's all his idea and you're the one feeling unsure. Remember that you can choose how far you want to go with strap-on sex as a fantasy. You don't have to penetrate him the first time, or ever if you decide you don't want to; you can decide to just "dip your toes" in the fantasy by wearing a strap-on during your regular sexual activities, or choose to wear it and playfully "threaten" him with it, but never use it unless you feel comfortable.

When you decide to make pegging a reality, it's up to you how far you want

> Remember that you can choose how far you want to go with strap-on sex as a fantasy.

to go—the possibilities for a man and a woman playing with a strap-on cock are endless, and the only limit is your imagination. What you do, and how you do it, depends on the type of fantasy the two of you may be enacting and what your comfort levels are in regard to pegging and anal play. The key here is to do what feels good, make it sexy, and stay within what's not embarrassing, distasteful, emotionally uncomfortable, physically harmful or dangerous for either of you. But at the same time, you'll both be fully mining the experience for its erotic potential, and having a blast while having some really hot sex—maybe even creating new masturbation material based on your real-life experiences.

Regardless of whose idea it is, you can ease into pegging by degrees, giving you space to figure out if you like wearing the cock or not. If it's your idea, you likely have all the fantasy components and details in your head, and all you need to do is tell him the key pieces. Pick out the main elements of what makes pegging hot for you—the sex act, the harness and dildo, a role such as dominant or submissive—and let him know exactly what in the fantasy turns you on.

A Man with a Plan: Talking Points for Him

Is this something you've always wanted to try, and now you've finally found the girl you'd like to do it with? Or have you been playing this way for a while with other partners, and now you'd like to get your desires out in the open with your current lover? Is this her idea, and you're like, *What's going on here?* Is this something you've both tried before and you'd like to try it again, or is it something you used to do together and now it's gone away and you'd like to bring it back?

For many men, strap-on sex is a favorite, dessert-like sex act that they spend much of their adult lives hoping to try, or trying to achieve with a variety of confused, squeamish, apprehensive—and sometimes lustily enthusiastic—partners. Men on the receiving side of the request, when she asks to wear the dick, will likely be feeling as confused and worried to varying degrees as a female partner might were he the one initiating the new sexual idea. The key here is—if you have questions about her intentions or feelings, ask them outright. And if you are requesting pegging, or asking for *more* pegging please, take the following suggestions into consideration.

Presenting a Case for Getting Pegged

- Asking for penetration is scary! Before you talk, think about how you might bring up the subject in a way that would feel safe for you: at home, after sex, before sex, in an intimate setting.
- There's never a perfectly "right time" to ask for something out of the ordinary sexually, though there are lots of "wrong" times. Don't bring it up when you're stressed or she's tired, when you're dealing with work or obligations—use your head for timing.
- You might feel more comfortable allowing a "third party" to spark the conversation—that third party being a book, movie, website, trip to a sex toy store or anything that mentions pegging.
- Make sure you use "I" statements, such as: "I'd like to see you in a strap-on more often," or "I'd get so turned on if I saw you wearing a strap-on," rather than "You never fuck me

anymore," or "You'd make me happier if you tried strap-on sex with me."

Consider ways in which you can encourage her to hear you out, and ask her to suspend judgment until you can explain why this is important, and how much fun you think the two of you can have with a strap-on. Be sure to reassure her that you find her incredibly sexy, and that this wouldn't be happening unless you felt safe to tell her your deepest desires. Your lover needs to hear that she is the star of your show, in addition to the fact that you're ready to become closer than you've ever been before.

> It could be the anal sex taboo, or even the forbidden quality of having a woman fuck you with a dildo that gets your pulse racing and your cock hard.

Ask her what she thinks and how she's feeling every chance you get—don't be afraid to guide the conversation so that you cover all the myths and fears in chapter 2. Hand her this book at any point, and be fearless when it comes to asking her what makes her reluctant point-blank. Be prepared for the conversation to have ups and downs, from everything to her wondering if she's enough for you, to her feeling like you want to just be "serviced," to her worries about your sexual orientation, or even just plain old poo-phobia.

Also, if you're on the requesting side of the conversation, be prepared to articulate your reasons why you love pegging, or why the idea sounds so appealing to you. It's likely a combination of fantasy, power exchange, taboo, physical sensations and being on the receiving end of such intimate nurturing. One

element will be guiding your desire above others. Perhaps it's
the power dynamic of her being in charge of something very
charged—penetration—that fuels your fires. Maybe it's the physical sensation alone: you'd like her to help you enjoy anal play,
or you'd like to share the experience—or experiment—with her.
Maybe this feels safer to you than trying it on your own.

It could be the anal sex taboo, or even the forbidden quality of having a woman fuck you with a dildo that gets your pulse
racing and your cock hard. You might just want a sexual experience where gender is playful or out of its typical roles; you
might relish the thought of her being stern and in control of
the sex, really putting you through something sexually, and yet
being sensitive and nurturing through the whole encounter.
Strap-on sex has many faces and many variations; understanding what excites you most about it will help you keep your
communication about your desires clear.

Three Lovers and a Dildo

Once you've broken the ice with strap-on play, you may want
to multiply your pleasure by inviting a third into your play; or,
perhaps a third playmate is the ingredient for making the introduction of strap-on sex a little easier. She might find her first-
time harness-wielding experience more palatable if she's trying
it out with another woman (while he watches), or it could be
that she'd feel comfortable under the tutelage of another woman
more experienced—with him getting pegged while she watches
or helps the extra (experienced) female partner. Another scenario might involve a couple with a second male who enjoys getting pegged, and serves as example and playmate for a novice

couple. Any of these ideas might make the experience more comfortable, and indeed quite hot. Because, of course, your pegging fantasies might revolve exclusively around a delicious strap-on threesome.

But how does one engineer more than two bodies coming together? A couple that adds an additional sex partner becomes a threesome, a combination that can express itself in a variety of ways, usually with two women and one man, or two men and one woman. It's essential that you think everything through and discuss your fears with your lover before you try a threesome. Think about exactly what it is you want to do in your fantasy scenario and what you don't want to do, and explore the possibilities of what could happen to upset you. Talk to your lover about all of it, and find out his or her concerns and perspectives as well. Jealousy is the main issue (outside of safe-sex considerations) that couples face when experimenting with threesomes and more, and it's the first thing you need to think about before trying any trysts. Even couples who have established trust over time and are deeply committed to each other encounter jealousy from time to time, and often unexpectedly.

Many couples make rules for their adventures with others, and set limits that keep both partners comfortable with the shared sex play. For instance, a woman might feel okay with a sexual encounter that includes another woman and her boyfriend, but set limits such as "no kissing," "no penis/vagina penetration," or "no oral sex." Others might make rules like "penetration is okay only if you're kissing me," "stay focused on me," "you can only touch him if you follow my instructions," or "only touch both of us at the same time." Think about what might upset you, and set your rules accordingly. Imagine your partner kissing another lover, and if it makes you feel bad, take that off the menu. Your comfort levels around images and sex acts will change over time, so don't feel like your rules are set in stone—they are for your partner, but you can change them if you feel good about it.

The inclusion of a third into your strap-on play can be a simple equation for a stable, grounded couple with clear communication, but it can also be like a minefield filled equally with danger and daisies. Read more about it in books such as my guidebook for fantasy-seeking couples *The Ultimate Guide to Sexual Fantasy* (with a variety of approaches from pickups to swinging), or if polyamory is your cup of lube, dive into Tristan Taormino's *Opening Up: A Guide to Polyamory.*

Chapter 8

First-Time Male
Anal Penetration

You've talked, you've rehearsed, you know all your lines...oh, wait. Okay, maybe you're not the star of the play on opening night, but it may feel like it before you get started. You'll both be aroused, excited and tingly about having a new sex style to play with—and so you might be a little nervous or apprehensive. That's exactly how you're supposed to feel, and with a few helpful suggestions and tips, you'll be focusing more on who comes first than how you're doing in no time.

The first time anyone goes near anyone else's butt, keep in mind the golden rules of anal penetration: start out aroused, go slow, use lots of lube, and talk about how fast or slow to go. Before strapping on a dildo and pillaging his village and storming his shores, you'll want to ease into anal penetration with your fingers first. Warming him up is the name of the game—and often, once he's warmed up, you'll be surprised at how his enjoyment takes over, making all those slow beginning steps of penetration seem like history.

Testing the Waters

First times have that funny catch-22 of being simultaneously scary and unforgettable. With a partner who is giving or receiving anal penetration for the first time, you'll want to be more support-ive than you would have ever thought necessary—patience, words of encouragement, slow pacing, and the willingness to stop at any time will help ensure a first time you'll want to remember.

Because you'll want to start out with him aroused, you'll likely be adding first anal contact to a sex act already in progress—like a blowjob, hand job or intercourse. Many men (though not all) enjoy penetration during fella-tio—that is, as long as you don't stop or interrupt the blowjob, nor should the contact on his cock stop when you first touch his anus, whatever the sex act in progress might be. You want a seamless transition to incor-porating anal contact into your fun.

> Keep in mind the golden rules of anal penetration: start out aroused, go slow, use lots of lube.

Fingers afford you the most feel-ing and movement, and that's what you'll want to touch his anus with first—and if you decide to go in, that is, if he responds positively like moaning assent or pushing back into your hand, fingers are what you'll always want to use first. You'll already have your hands on him caressing and adding to your sexual encounter, and when he's turned on you can experiment with massaging his buttocks and caressing the crack between his cheeks. If he responds positively, try slowly sliding a finger over the opening to his anus while you're stroking his cock.

Be sure your hands are clean (read: scrubbed—no dirt or grime under your nails) and your fingernails are trimmed and filed smooth. Make sure you don't have any tiny cuts or hang-nails. Many women like to use latex or nitrile (nonlatex) gloves for anal contact and penetration. It makes for a perfectly smooth surface (for him), keeps your hands clean, and is a clean surface to introduce into the rectum (minimal bacteria). Best of all, gloves can be removed when soiled, to reveal a clean, bacteria-free hand that can play in other areas.

Anal Penetration Rules! I Mean, Rules

- Only insert fingers, a plug or the strap-on dildo when he's already really turned on.
- Never use a toy without a flared base.
- Don't insert items that can create a dangerous vacuum, like bottles.
- Use lots and lots of lube. Anal tissue is thin, does not lubricate itself, and can tear easily.
- If it hurts you're either going too fast, you need more lube, the item is too big, or he's not really in the mood right then.
- Go slow: very, very slow.

His Concerns: Staying Hard and Keeping Clean

Contrary to popular conceptions, men's erections and orgasms don't erupt like Old Faithful. Nothing in the male or female pleasure cycle is entirely predictable, and that goes for arousal, orgasm, ejaculation, the timing involved for any of it, and especially erection. Erections work on two levels simultaneously. One is the physical: touching your genitals or an erogenous zone, or having them touched, triggers a response along nerve pathways to begin the flow of blood into your penis. The other level is the path that leads directly from your brain: an image, fantasy, idea, or mental or visual stimulus triggers the same nerve response, filling your penis with blood and growing it into an erection. The stiffest cocks and the hottest sex come when both pathways are stimulated at the same time.

The perplexing thing about erections is that they sometimes like to come and go as they please. They arrive at the party uninvited or leave when everyone's having fun. During strap-on sex his may stiffen and soften as his pleasure cycle dips and peaks along its normal course—don't take it personally if he loses his hard-on when you play with his ass, but ask him if he's enjoying himself to make sure it's cool to proceed. Chances are high that hard-on will return, and if it doesn't, it's no big deal if he's enjoying the sex play. Don't forget that age, anxiety, stress, or medication can sometimes make erections altogether unreliable.

Of course, medication might be just the thing to alleviate concern about erections; a good number of adventurous men might add erection meds like Cialis (Tadalafil), Levitra (Vardenafil) or Viagra (Sildenafil) to the mix. Available by prescription (or online, and at your own risk), erection pills like Cialis and Viagra serve to maintain erections by increasing genital blood flow and acting on the circulatory system (Tadalafil relaxes blood vessels in the penis, thereby increasing blood flow and aiding in erection). Which is why you should only use such cock candies under the advice of a doctor; they can have adverse or even serious side effects, especially for men with cardiovascular risk factors—Viagra is also used to treat pulmonary arterial hypertension. With any of these drugs, it's important to remember that they don't work "cold," meaning that the user needs to already be at least slightly aroused or in the mood for the pills to work. They won't make you aroused if you're not already; but when they do work, it can be quite a night of hard cock and intense anal pleasure, where he might "wear out" before his hard-on does.

He's probably not just worrying about what his penis is up to (or not), as it's even more likely he's concerned about what his ass looks like, and whether or not he's "clean" back there. Asses look like—asses! They're fuzzy, differently colored than the rest of the body; they have a whimsical-yet-unsettling winking eye, the reminder of waste leaving the body—they are in many ways one of the things that make us most human. Certainly, they make us humble.

The stiffest cocks and the hottest sex come when both pathways—physical and mental—are stimulated at the same time.

The best way to overcome cleanliness fears is to shower or take a bath beforehand, though that's not always possible. But if you both do opt to bathe in preparation, feel free to flirt with his ass in the shower, cleaning and massaging it a bit in the soap-and-water sanctuary of the bathroom. Some people like to take an enema before anal sex, though it isn't necessary.

At any given time there is nothing in the rectum—if he's healthy and doesn't have loose stools for whatever reasons, generally there is little matter in the anus to discover with a dildo. But it's naïve to think that there's absolutely nothing in there at all, so realistically, know that you may encounter a bit of material, which often reveals itself when you notice the lube becoming discolored, most often after the fun is over. Sometimes you will come in contact with a bit of fecal matter—or rather, your dildo will. That's the reality of anal play; if it happens, be sensitive and cool and move along. Unscented "baby wipes" are an ace to have up your sleeve for cleanup, and come in really handy if he wants to be sure he's clean but there isn't time (or the availability) of a shower or bidet. The best advice for avoiding a fouled dildo is for him to go to the bathroom shortly before you start playing, to be sure all is evacuated.

The Right Lube

In chapter 10 I'll explain how to pick the right dildo, harness and even the right scenario for starting your strap-on adventures, but don't even think about going anywhere near anyone's butt, ever, without lube. Moreover, it should be the lube that's right for both of you, suitable for the toy you're playing with (be it dildo or finger), and even the mood you're both in. Take my word for it—lube not only makes for a safe encounter, it's how you make it all feel so amazingly good.

If you've never tried lube for sex at all, I insist that you buy a bottle immediately and see what you've been missing. Even if you think you don't need it, try it anyway, because you'll want to experiment with how it feels before you go slathering it on any synthetic appendages intended for the back door. For anal play lube is an absolute requirement, but the way lube makes slippery genitals even more slippery is a sensation that has to be experienced to really be appreciated. *Yum.*

Lube comes in a range of thicknesses, consistencies, flavors and styles. Finding the lube that's right for you will be a matter of personal preference, though some people like different lubes for different activities, much like a cook will use different seasonings for different dishes. Many sex educators recommend thick gel-like lubes for anal sex, but not all users agree. Start with a sample pack, or a thick gel and a lighter formula to see what feels right. You may prefer a lube that is more like a long-lasting lotion, like Liquid Silk. Or a thicker gel-like lube such as Astrogel or Maximus may do the trick and have the staying power you need—especially for fitting big things in (ahem) small spaces. You might prefer the oil-like feel and forever-lasting, waterproof qualities of silicone-based lubes like Eros, or Wet silicone formulas. Just be careful not to use silicone lubricants with toys made of silicone material—most often, these two don't get along and silicone lube has ruined the surface of many a good silicone dick, rendering an expensive, often favorite, toy useless.

Water-based lubes—including silicone—are the standard, as they clean up easily with water and are safe to use around latex (like gloves and condoms). Read the ingredients list before you use any lube, if you're at all sensitive—colorings, additives and flavors can have undesirable effects, like irritation and allergy stimulation. Never, ever use a lubricant with Nonoxynol-9 (a detergent spermicide), as the ingredient has been shown to cause more harm to tissues and membranes than its purported good: it was marketed originally as an HIV preventative, but studies revealed it actually abrades skin, leaving users irritated and more susceptible to viruses than before use.

Never, ever use lubes like Anal-Eze. Lubricants with benzocaine and numbing agents such as Anal-Eze, "Good Head Gel," and desensitizing creams contain oils, flavors and colorings, and are very unsafe. Numbing the back of your throat, the penis, the vagina, and especially the anus can lead to serious injury and infections that can (and often do) land users in the doctor's office or ER. Think: you can't feel the skin breaking or tearing, and if it's the anus, there are fecal bacteria. When you can't feel pain, you are getting injured, period.

Lots of people ask about flavored lubes for analingus (rimming), and they're great for anal-oral contact, but you should switch to a more functional lube for penetration. Flavored lubricants are a fun treat, and readily available at any adult toy or novelty store. They actually don't taste very good; imagine the flavor of lube mixed with artificial flavoring and sweetener. *Yum!* The pictures on the labels look much better than the products taste—and you may want to ask yourself what you do (or don't) want to taste, anyway. Edibles come in two categories: lubricants that are water-based and edible gels, liquids, or sprays that may contain oils. No matter how completely you think you are licking it off, even the smallest amount of oil can cause a condom, dental dam, or glove to break.

That's not to say that licking something yummy off of your lover isn't fun—it is. It can be a treat to have a little something extra to lick, something that makes your strokes longer and more focused. The water-based brand ID Juicy Lube has by far the cleanest ingredient list, no artificial coloring, and the largest selection of flavors; I recommend sticking with their line of fruit flavors, though I admit Bubblegum Blast is a favorite. Hot Licks is a super-sugary tasting line of water-based flavored gels that heat up when you breathe on them (though the heating-up sensation isn't for everyone), and they come in flavors like strawberry and cinnamon. Kama Sutra sells a whole range of products made for licking off excited body parts, and their Oil of Love also heats up, but keep in mind that many of their products contain trace amounts of oil.

If you're not worried about safe-sex gear, you're more than welcome to use oil-based lubes for anal penetration, and many people go no further than their kitchen for anal lube—but keep in mind that oils

> It can be a treat to have a little something extra to lick, something that makes your strokes longer and more focused.

retain bacteria and are not the most sanitary thing to insert into someone's colon. There are a whole lot of lubes that feel oily (like silicone lubes) that are a lot safer, and peace of mind goes a long way with a sex act that requires so much trust and a focus on safety in the first place. Plus, not everyone wants an ass that smells like Crisco.

First Penetration

As the sexual activity continues, you'll want to turn up the volume on your anal explorations. With the flat of your finger, or fingers, press lightly on the opening and hold it there. Increase the pressure a little, massaging and pressing in circular motions. Go very slowly, and listen to his cues or verbal instructions—for some guys, simply having their anus touched is all it takes to push them over the edge. Pay attention to lubrication, reapply more frequently than you think necessary, and never rely solely on saliva—it's not up to the job. In porn films they make it look like that's all they use, but that's not the case—they just don't show you the anal suppositories and numerous applications of lube.

Move your flattened fingers in a circular motion, and begin experimenting with penetration by pressing one well-lubed finger at the base of the opening (toward his tailbone). Massage the opening's base, and ask him if he wants you to go farther. Slowly slide your finger in up to the first joint (about an inch), and hold it there for a few breaths. You'll feel the ring of muscles around his opening squeeze and contract—just stay still as the muscles relax.

When you feel his muscles relax, slide your finger in slowly a little bit more, then back out, doing a gentle in-and-out, not all the way in yet. Once again, this may be all it takes for him to come, or to decide that it's not what he wants right now—but if he does want more, following his directions and body language from here, you can progress to more stimulation. Many men like it if you stroke their penises (hard or soft) in time with your thrusting finger. Keep in mind that what feels like little movements to you will feel like huge movements to him—err on the side of small thrusts and shallow penetration unless he directs you otherwise.

Feel with your fingers whether or not the skin of his anus is "dragging" on your fingers or glove; add more lube to be sure this doesn't happen. If you want to add lube with your finger still in place, back it out a little, drizzle lubricant on the visible part of your finger, and massage it inward. You can go deeper or faster, or even add more fingers—but the most important thing is to do everything so slowly that you almost can't stand the wait. Anal penetration hurts when you go too fast, you don't use enough lube, the recipient isn't relaxed, or he doesn't really want to be doing it.

How to Stimulate the Spot

There's anal stimulation, and there's prostate stimulation, and strap-on sex is where the two sensations become greater together. Of course penetration is the most direct way to stimulate the prostate, but direct prostate stimulation with fingers differs slightly from prostate stimulation via rubber cock, because you focus your attention on the gland rather than on the fullness, pressure, or rhythm you're applying to his anus.

When he's aroused and ready for penetration, take the necessary steps to pleasurably insert your finger, then slightly curve it toward the front of his body: facing him (perhaps with his penis in your mouth or other hand), make a come-hither stroking motion with your finger. Don't poke, push, or stab forward. The gland is delicate, and, as we saw earlier, because of its positioning, some men report the sensation of having to pee when it's stimulated. That's a feeling that some men don't like at all, and you may wind up switching activities if he's uncomfortable. If he experiences any pain when his prostate is touched, he should have it checked by his doctor.

At this point, you can massage his prostate and penis in tandem to orgasm if you like—if he likes, too!

Chapter 9

More Male Anal Foreplay

M anual stimulation—fingering him—is a sublime way to get him in the mood for pegging, or can even be the main event itself. But don't think you need to stop there when you're having fun—easing up to (or teasing him with the inevitability of) strap-on sex has many options, from rimming to butt plugs and beyond.

Rimming

Rimming, or analingus, is kissing, caressing, or penetrating your lover's anal opening with your tongue. For many people, rimming is a delicious experience, on both the giving and the receiving end. Some say there is nothing as arousing as having their lover's warm, soft tongue and lips give them pleasure in such an incredibly intimate place, and those who love to give it find the experience equally arousing. Also, the feeling of doing something taboo or "dirty" heightens the experience for some. Because the delicate pucker of the anus is packed with sensitive nerve endings, rimming can be all it takes to push someone over the orgasmic edge.

For men, rimming adds a new spectrum of pleasure to the sexual experience. A fantastic blowjob can include delicate licks and flutters of the tongue on and around the anus, and rimming can be a great introduction to the sensation of anal penetration. For men who enjoy being penetrated, this is a delicious tease for the main course to come, and for men who aren't sure about penetration, rimming allows them to comfortably try out the sensation of anal stimulation to see if they might like it.

> With the delicate pucker of the anus in full view, gently kiss and lick his cheeks.

The easiest position for rimming is doggy-style, with the rim-ee on all fours. This lets you gently spread his cheeks with your hands, and see everything clearly as you dip your tongue in and out. If he has a lot of hair down there, this position is optimal for parting the furry seas—and if this notion makes you uncomfortable, let it be known that *everyone* has hair down there. If you do not naturally have hair around your anus, you are either a) too young to be reading this, b) shaving or waxing it, or c) a genetic anomaly. Doggy-style licking is ideal because it also provides a fantastic rear view of his testicles, which you can squeeze, rub, and pull on as you lick. Also, you can pull his erect penis back between his legs for reverse cocksucking, though some men find this uncomfortable. When in doubt, ask how it feels.

With the delicate pucker of the anus in full view, gently kiss and lick his cheeks as they slope inward toward the crack. Work your way closer into the furrow, taking your time to let him get used to the sensation—or to tease him if you know he likes it. You can make your first touch in various ways:

- Lick the entire furrow from top to bottom as you would an ice-cream cone, with a big, flat tongue.
- With softened lips, kiss it directly, over and over.
- Press your flattened tongue against the opening and hold it, then slowly start to move it in with an up and down motion, or give him an in-and-out massage.
- With the very tip of your tongue, lightly lick in a ring around the rim of the opening—"rimming" him.

You can start with one of these and then try them all out to see what he likes. When you find something that makes him moan, groan, and push his butt in your face, stay with it for a few minutes. Gradually, work your tongue into a rhythm with a short, firm lick. Continue the beat for a while: this should get him pretty aroused. If you decide you want to go a step further, begin darting your tongue in as you lick, graduating to what's called "tongue-fucking." Moan your appreciation and see how he responds—moaning vibrates your tongue and simulates a vibrator. When you want him to explode, slide a lubed hand onto his cock and jack him off while you lick—there's no sensation in the world like it.

Adding Sex Toys

Once he's anally warmed up and ready for more penetration, you can bring sex toys into the picture. Vibrators will feel fantastic on his ass, and you can tease and penetrate him while

Vibrators will feel fantastic on his ass, and you can tease and penetrate him while you suck, stroke or fuck him.

you suck, stroke or fuck him. The thing to know about vibrators and anal stimulation is that the outer third of the anus, and the prostate, contain more nerve endings than the anal canal and respond best to touch and vibration. The inner portion, inside the canal, has fewer nerve endings near the skin's surface and responds to feelings of fullness, pressure, and rhythm.

So, a vibrator will feel intense (intensely good) around the opening and the prostate area. But the vibration won't be a factor deep inside—the size, shape, and motion of the vibe will. To maximize your buzz, select insertable vibrators that have the vibration located at the base. When bringing a vibe into the action, start on the lowest speed, and give him more as he asks for it.

Squirt liberal amounts of lube on any toy you use, and reapply frequently. You can fuck the daylights out of him anally with a dildo he likes. Or, insert a butt plug and keep it in place while you bring him to orgasm; just don't leave it in for extended periods, or it will get uncomfortable.

More Manual Stimulation: Butt Plugs and Beads

Butt plugs are typically nonvibrating bullet-shaped toys with a flat, flared base made to insert in the anus during different kinds of sex play, and are intended to stay put. However, this isn't always what happens—smaller plugs, when properly lubed up for insertion, tend to come out (or shoot out) when the invol-

untary muscles of the anal sphincter contract and relax, especially at the point of orgasm; if you like, you can hold it in place
with your free hand. But most butt plugs are created in the ideal
shape to stay put; a wide base and narrow "neck" make them
ideal toys for hands-free anal penetration, and a lasting feeling
of fullness during other activities, such as oral sex, penetration
or hand jobs. Because they're made to stay put, anal plugs with
a narrow neck and bulbous top aren't great for in-and-out thrusting, as the stress of opening and closing the anal muscles tends
to feel uncomfortable, especially if you are sensitive to anal pain.
If it hasn't been forced out during orgasm—if it's big and stays
in place—after he comes ask him to take a few deep breaths
and let him know you are going to remove the plug on an
exhale—then remove it on the second or third exhale.

Remember, sex toys safe for anal penetration have a flared
base: this prevents them from being pulled into the anal canal,
where they can get lost, as we saw in chapter 5. Not all toys
sold for anal use are actually safe to put in your butt; be a sex-
smart shopper.

Anal beads are basically a knotted string with plastic beads
every inch or so, with a large ring at the end that functions as
a handle. Not all anal beads are created equal, and quality ranges
from cheap plastic to metal and precious gems; some versions
are beaded wands, rather than strings. Like all butt toys, anal
beads should be carefully examined before use. If using the string
version, make sure all the knots are secure. Plastic beads are
made in factories and the beads themselves often have sharp
seams—file any ridges or seams down with a nail file to ensure
a smooth set of beads. Make sure your handle is secure, and check
the base of any "stringless" varieties for strength.

The Aneros (which can be found at malegspot.com) is an anal plug made specifically for prostate massage. Unlike most plugs for guys, the Aneros was painstakingly researched to come up with the very best design for easy insertion and hands-free prostate massage. The thinking behind its anatomically correct design is that contraction of the sphincter muscles provides the rhythm for orgasmic release, and the creators claim that male multiple orgasms are possible with correct use of their toy. The Aneros comes in a variety of sizes. It is exceptionally smooth, white, and has a shape that looks fanciful but slides in easily and stays put once it's in. The curved shape allows prostate stimulation with the slightest squeeze of his pelvic muscles, or you can massage the prostate pleasurably with a rocking motion using the curled handle. Whether or not claims of male multiples are true, the Aneros has a loyal following and is a darling of the sex toy boutique scene. If you're feeling adventurous, it's highly recommended.

Picture Perfect

ALISON TYLER

MY CONDO IS ON THE TOP FLOOR of a very tall, very posh building on Wilshire Boulevard. I bought it because of the view. From one side of the living room, you can see the glittering lights of Beverly Hills and downtown L.A. From the balcony on the other side, you can almost see all the way to the ocean. At night, the city is a shimmering carpet.

I am above it all.

When I first brought Nicholas home, he was stunned. He spent hours on the balcony looking out at Los Angeles. It *is* beautiful from high up, regardless of what L.A.-bashers may say. It's an amazing metropolis when you don't have to go down and get involved with the traffic, and the noise, and the chaos.

Nicholas spent so much time on the balcony and in the living room looking out of the floor-to-ceiling windows that we began to play there, as well. My bedroom was all but forgotten. Our lovemaking occurred on the black leather sofa, on the dark scarlet rug, or spread out on the wooden coffee table I picked up in an antique store on Melrose.

Because we were in this new environment, we somehow felt freer with each other. Freer to explore; to use new toys, new tools; to discover the wide range of sensations available outside of a bedroom.

First, and most basic, was the luxury of making love on the rug. I spread my boy out on the floor, with the soft rug tickling

his ass from below and my tongue stroking him from above. I
loved the way his body looked against the ruby red of the expensive fabric. There was something so base about screwing on the
floor rather than on a mattress. It was as if we simply couldn't
control ourselves, couldn't manage to walk the twenty steps
down the hall to the bedroom. I loved that.

We lit candles on the mantel and a fire in the fireplace and
fucked by their light alone. His pale skin glowed in the light
from the many candles, and the intensely colorful tattoos that
snaked around his arms and along his flat stomach seemed to
come alive. I traced my fingertips over the vibrant designs, traced
my tongue over the art of his body. He let me play however I
wanted to. Of course he did, because our relationship is defined
by power and rules. I am in power, and I make the rules. Soon,
I had Nicholas tied down on the rug, his wrists cuffed and
anchored to the leg of the sofa, his ankles captured with the
leather thongs. Fastened, and spread wide apart. I blindfolded
him with one of my favorite silk scarves and brought over a candle
from the mantel. A special candle I'd chosen ahead of time for
this particular purpose.

Slowly, I dripped the wax over his naked skin, watching him
squirm and twist. I enjoyed the spectacle, and I continued to
make pinpoint drops around his hard nipples, then worked my
way down that sensual plane of his concave stomach to his tender
inner thighs. And then, when the wax had cooled and hardened,
I brought my mouth to the same spots and licked and lapped
at them, confusing him with the warring sensations.

I could tell that he liked it. How could I not? His cock was
at full mast by the time I finished trailing my tongue from wax
drip to wax drip. And although I would have loved to deep-throat

him until I swallowed every drop of his sweet juices, I wanted more. I wanted to take him higher, to take him further. But breaking away was too difficult. Nicholas needed the release. He moaned and tried to spread his legs wider apart, but they were as far open as they could be.

I knew what that meant. He wanted me to lick his balls. "Say it," I insisted.

He turned his head toward my voice, eyes still shaded by the blindfold.

"Tell me what you want." Yeah, I knew, but hearing the words would turn me on like nothing else.

"Please, Amanda," he groaned. "Please. Lick them. Get them all wet."

I did just what he said. I sucked his balls into my mouth, lapped them with my tongue. Sure, I might be in charge when we fuck, but that doesn't mean I won't reward him. Yet as soon as I sensed he was about to shoot, I pulled back.

Quickly undoing his ankles, I had him roll over on the carpet. He did so gingerly, moving his hips carefully because of his raging hard-on. I spanked his ass for him, using only my bare hand, but working him hard, nonetheless. The firelight lit his reddening asscheeks, adding to the warmth of the glow. I gave him twenty decent strokes until he was breathing hard and squirming. He was hot from the spanking, but had not nearly reached his pinnacle for pain.

Without a word of warning, I freed Nicholas's still-cuffed wrists from the sofa leg, and helped him to stand. Then I led him to the far wall in the room, basking in the fact that he trusted me. He didn't question where I was taking him, didn't try to pull away. That faith made me crave him all the more.

I have a large, heavy painting on this wall, which I removed. The hook was high enough in the wall that, once I looped the handcuff chain over it, Nicholas had to stand on tiptoes. It's a sturdy hook—the picture that usually hangs on the wall is an impressive one with a thick, wooden frame. I knew from experience that it would be able to hold my latest acquisition: Nicholas.

Next, I took a heavy belt from one of my leather coats, doubled it, and gave his ass a proper hiding. *That* got the reaction I was looking for. Pretty stripes decorated his firm, naked buttocks, and when I reached forward, I could feel how rock solid his cock had become. His erection felt as if it had been poured from plaster.

But I wasn't done.

Far from it.

With Nicholas so well mounted, I pressed my body to his back. I am tall in bare feet, but in my five-inch heels I'm just about the same height as Nicholas. I let him feel that I was packing, and he groaned and tried to press himself up against the cool wall, searching for relief.

But there was no relief. Not yet.

I split my slacks and set my toy free, then slid off the blindfold and made Nicholas turn his head to watch me as I lubed myself up. I wanted him to admire my cock. I wanted him to dream about where that cock was going to go.

"In your ass," I said, watching his handsome young face. "Deep inside of your ass. I know you like to fuck *me* there. And now it's your turn."

He looked as if he'd never blink again, he was focused so intently on the way my hand moved piston-smooth on my synthetic cock. I could tell that he was mesmerized by the motion of my fist against the plastic, and as I lubed up, I started to feel as if the toy had become part of me. As if I might actually shoot my own load if I worked myself hard enough.

Wouldn't that have been lovely?

But what I really wanted was to be inside Nicholas, and I told him that.

"This is for you, Nicky-boy. *All* for you. I'm going to slip it in slowly, so you can really feel it. I'm going to work every last inch into your asshole and then press my body against yours, so that I'm driving in deep, as far as I can go. That's what you want, isn't it?"

Nicholas's face turned pink as I spoke, but I could tell from the look in his dark green eyes how ready he was.

Still, I needed to hear him say the words.

"Isn't it?" I murmured, now leaning right up against him.

"Yes, Amanda," he said, practically choking on the words.

Oh, how I loved the sound of his voice. He was desperate. He wanted me to fuck him, and he could hardly wait for the first fierce jolt of my body on his. Quickly, I used my greased-up fingertips to lube his hole, and then I was in—driving hard from the start, gratified to hear the moans of pleasure escaping immediately from his lips. It was clear to me that he loved the way this felt. Loved the feeling of my still-clothed body against his totally naked one. There was no doubt about who was in charge here. No question at all.

I fucked him until I came, the pressure of the dildo pressing against my swollen clit, making my orgasm spiral through me. Hungrily, I dug my fingers into his back, clawing out every last bit of my pleasure. Nicholas lowered his head at the sensation and let go, decorating the wall with his own come.

He looked embarrassed as I let him down, embarrassed as I set him free. But when I undid his wrists, *he* was the one to come forward, to take the harness off for me, to kiss me between my thighs and whisper how amazing the encounter had been for him.

"Fucking good," he sighed, "so damn good."

We hung the picture back up on the wall together. But I have a good feeling we'll be using that hook again soon. You see, Nicholas is my favorite piece of art. He's picture perfect.

Chapter 10

Harnesses and Dildos

Y ou can be as ready and rarin' to go a-pegging as you like—
you've read the manuals, done your communication
troubleshooting, you've even had first contact, like in those alien
movies. But in order to make strap-on sex really happen in all
of its hottest permutations you need to do one essential thing:
go shopping!

You'll need the right gear to make your pegging adventures
sing the dulcet tones of sweet, penetrative pleasure. That means
selecting a strap-on harness form the oodles of models to choose
from, getting the right dildo—or dildos, as you'll likely want
more than one size—and any other accessories to make your
strap-on fantasies come true. Accessories can include vibes for
in-harness clitoral stimulation, sleeves that make for simulta-
neous penetration, and even clever double dildos that thrust in
and out of both of you in time with your gyrating endeavors.
Oh—and don't forget the lube!

Strap-Ons: Shopping and Selection

Shopping for strap-ons together is an experience many couples find to be a sort of intellectual foreplay. Together, you assess your options and let your imaginations run wild. Would she look better in a black leather harness or a red vinyl sparkly number with shiny silver buckles? Considering the myriad function options on harnesses, deciding on that detail can be pretty hot, too—do you want one that leaves her "open" for genital access, or one that you know will rub her clit when she's thrusting?

Where you shop is important, especially if you want quality toys that will be hygienic and worth the money, perform as expected and last more than a few encounters. There are many suggestions for places to shop for strap-on gear online and off in the last chapter of this book, with advice on every front. Read that chapter carefully before you visit a store, and definitely before you pull out your wallet for an online transaction.

Would she look better in a black leather harness or a red vinyl sparkly number with shiny silver buckles?

When choosing a strap-on, take into account what kind of strap-on fantasy scenario you have in mind—pretty much any fantasy can be realized if you know the limitations of the market and how to get around them.

Newcomers to strap-on play will want to make their first purchase an inexpensive harness made of fabric or nylon and a one-off rubber dildo in a pleasing and reasonable shape. Options for harnesses range from neoprene and nylon to glittery vinyl, rubber, see-through plastic, leather and velvet. Many online retailers have beginners' strap-on kits, though I suggest you purchase these from reputable (non-novelty) retailers so you get a quality product that will actually do what it's supposed to, even if it's inexpensive.

All too often, novelty toy retailers will sell badly constructed, mass-produced harnesses made out of fabric and elastic straps, which tend to fit terribly, have the dildo rest in the wrong place, and, often, involve elastic straps so loose the dildo winds up doing embarrassing things when you're trying to thrust, pull out, and repeat. A good harness will have a solid method of attachment, as in straps with wide elastic, or leather or nylon straps with buckles or D-rings so you can tighten the harness to your body.

Harnesses come in two general styles: a single-strap that is worn like a G-string panty and two-strap models, which have two straps running from the pubic bone, along the crease between the inner thigh and genitals, and underneath the buttocks to attach to the waistband in back. Some prefer the G-string style, saying it's a very stable base for the dildo and that it rubs the clit nicely when the wearer is thrusting; others complain of "buttcrack rash" from the center string rubbing on their anus and tailbone. Another complaint about the G-string style is that it limits access to the wearer's genitals, so if a girl wanted to be penetrated or to massage her clit, it would be difficult. Also, they're not adaptable for male wearers.

A girl can jack off her cock with one hand or get a blowjob, while rubbing her clit or fucking herself with another dildo at the same time.

Two-strap harnesses allow for plenty of genital access so the wearer (of any gender) can masturbate or penetrate herself, or be penetrated by another, while wearing the harness. For instance, a girl can jack off her cock with one hand or get a blowjob, while rubbing her clit or fucking herself with another dildo at the same time—increasing her chances of fulfilling the fantasy of coming "with her cock."

You'll also face choices when selecting a harness as to how the dildo is attached to or worn in the harness. Some strap-ons will have a simple hole in the middle where the dildo is pulled through from the inside; while these are the easiest to get dildos in and out of, it's a "one size fits most" hole that will have smaller dildos sliding around and make bigger dildos difficult (or impossible) to squeeze in. A harness with a hole is especially suited for dildo and harness manufacturer Vixen's unique double dildos that penetrate both partners at once with the thrusting of the harness. More versatile harnesses have four straps that come through a triangle-shaped base and attach to a removable rubber O-ring in the center. This style provides the most stable base for a dildo, period, and different O-ring sizes are available for purchase (many of these harnesses ship with three ring sizes), and cleanup is a snap.

Website Stockroom.com has a very specialized harness called the Double Penetration Harness, just for men who want to wear a harness to provide double penetration to their female partners. Of course he doesn't need to be hard when he wears it; this specialty harness really just makes it a lot more comfortable for a guy to wear an extra cock while having space for his own (attached) cock and balls to hang while he fucks his girlfriend (or anyone else, for that matter). It's essentially a single-strap nylon harness with a cock ring for the wearer's penis and testicles (providing a constriction that some men find pleasurable and that may help maintain an erection longer), with another ring just above it for the dildo.

You'll find that harnesses come in a wide variety of shapes, styles and sizes and can be tailored to fit virtually any fantasy scenario you and your lover have in mind. Strap-ons are for women, men and transpeople of all genders and orientations who want a little (or a big) something extra in their pants.

The material you choose for your strap-on is up to you; I prefer leather for warmth and appearance, and buckles for no-slip fastening, but for travel and getting through airports you might want a fabric or neoprene model; these are machine washable, which is very nice for cleanup. Leather should always be cleaned according to leather care instructions (search online or follow manufacturer's care instructions), and rubber, plastic and PVC strap-ons can be cleaned with an antibacterial wipe-down.

How Your Strap-On Should Fit

If you're shopping online you won't get a sense of how your strap-on is going to fit you, nor will you be able to ask questions about function and comfort—and no one will tell you that strap-ons are worn lower than you might think. When you try on a harness for the first time, it feels a little weird—until you understand that it's designed to hold the dildo at precisely the same spot as a penis sits on a man's pubic bone. When you first slip into it, you'll likely think that it's too low, like a pair of low-rise jeans, rather than a standard pair of Levi's. However, that's exactly how it's supposed to fit, and once you tighten down the straps, you'll get a sense of the pubic snugness required to make a stable base for your new dildo, and also a feeling for how your pubic bone will provide the foundation for your thrusting.

Slip into your harness alone before you actually use it, so you can get familiar with the way it fits, how to tighten it, and how it looks and feels. The straps should be tight enough to withstand thrusting, but not so tight they pinch or cut into your skin; give the dildo a few tugs to see how it feels. The dildo shouldn't slip out, or slide around too much (though a little movement is fine). The dildo should rest right on or just above your pubic bone; if you worry about it getting sore from thrusting, you can buy a specially made pad of thin foam to cushion your pubic bone.

Hooray for Dildos

While it's important to get the right harness, it's equally important to get the right dildo. If you're just testing the waters on this whole pegging thing, you'll want to start out with an inexpensive, small model—that way you don't wind up with a toy that's too big for a nervous boyfriend, nor will you be out serious cash if you both decide that pegging isn't for you. You can spend serious money on nice dildos, but that's something you'll only want to do if you know you're going to try this more than once, or if money is no object and you'd like to ride in a Mercedes the first time around, rather than a sensible economy compact.

My recommendation is actually that you get two dildos for your first purchase if you can; it's difficult to judge size and shape until you actually get to play with a dildo and see how it fits (in him, and your harness), and with two you have the option of trading up or down in size depending on how he's feeling about what's in his butt. If it's too much, trade down; if he's greedy, give him more. Everyone's happy!

Shopping for dildos to play with other women may also have you buying more than one cock; whereas with beginning male anal penetration you'll want to be sure at least one of your choices is a small, smooth model, with another woman you'll want to get a couple different sizes as not all women are going to have a "one size fits all" approach to what size and shape dildo they want to be penetrated with. Of course, shopping together is ideal; at the very least find out beforehand if she has preferences on size (big, thick, thin, short) or shape (realistic, ridged, dolphin-shaped).

Before you shop for dicks, know what you're looking for. A dildo is basically defined as any penetrative, nonvibrating device—but aside from the clinical definition of what makes a dildo *not* a vibrator, dildos comprise a vast category of wonderful, whimsical, bizarre and sometimes scary penetration toys. Dildos in garden-variety porn shops are mostly marketed for vaginal and female anal penetration (unless you shop in a gay porn shop, with its miles of molded rubber gay porn star cock just looking to go home with the right man), and they can all be used for wonderfully intense mock blowjobs, especially when worn in a strap-on harness.

Before you shop for dicks, know what you're looking for.

In general, there are two styles of dildo: representational and nonrepresentational. Representational is a loose term here, as even the most realistic dildos tend to look like bizarrely colored doll parts, though the dildo manufacturing industry is where some of the more incredible innovations have occurred in prosthetic realism—most notably with Vixen Creations' incredibly realistic feeling silicone Tex dildo (made with VixSkin™). But representational dildos all usually look penile in shape, whereas nonrepresentational dildos can be anything from smooth shafts in pearlescent turquoise, to mermaids or bumpy sculpted figurative works of art.

Some dildos have a suction-cup base, allowing the user to stick them on smooth surfaces like bathroom tile or the side of a tub, or even a hard bar stool. Dildos made for harness use have a flared, flat base so they fit into the harness base, and these dildos are also suitable for safe anal use as the flared base can be used as a handle to retrieve the toy. They're also great for practicing deep-throat fellatio, as you can again use the base as a handle as you explore the comfort zone of your gag reflex. Extra-long dildos (and double dildos) are great for when you need a little extra reach, when you have mobility issues or wrist injuries, or when a long handle makes penetration more comfortable. Or, of course, when you like really deep penetration.

Selecting the best dildo for male anal penetration will of course be up to him, but I recommend getting a dildo that is not contoured, bumpy or wider at the base than the top. Pick a smooth, slender dildo for your first strap-on adventures. The sphincter muscles are a ring about one-half inch in depth, and wide-based dildos put uncomfortable stress on the (possibly already tense and worried) muscles by stretching them on the "in" thrust. A bulb at the end is fine, and can be helpful for prostate stimulation, but remember you'll then be putting the biggest part in first, which might be too intense for your virgin.

Advanced Toys

How about strap-on sex, no harness required? Companies like woman-owned Tantus (tantussilicone.com) thought long and hard (and *long*, and *hard*) to come up with a design for a dildo that can be worn by a female partner for hands-free penetration without a harness, and they came up with the Feeldoe. It really works, and there are legions of happy product testers behind the final design they came up with, which is a bulb that fits snugly inside the vagina, with a right-angle penis-shaped shaft extending out the front. It comes in different sizes, is made of silicone, and some models come with a vibrator at the base situated for clitoral stimulation and vibration during penetration. The shaft is a nice smooth shape for anal penetration, as it's not contoured. The small one is my recommendation for novice ass-tronauts.

Double dildos crafted in a similar style but created for use with or without a harness are Vixen Creations' (vixencreations.com) Nexus and Nexus Jr. Tired of standard double dildos that are essentially a stick with two insertable ends difficult to manipulate in tandem for orgasm, they wanted to make a double that *really* worked. They did; the silicone Nexus is a boomerang-shaped double with one shorter, slightly curved end, and a longer straighter end that allows true in-and-out motions for both users. It also works quite well when worn in a harness (with a hole for insertion) so both lovers can enjoy more controlled penetration and thrusting, and some clever users have even used button-fly jeans in lieu of a harness with this versatile toy.

So, how about those classic double dildos? They do indeed work for penetration, and are an awful lot of fun to play with, even if they may not work as well as you'd expect for penetrative orgasms. But they don't work the way they do in porn movies, where even the slightest motion brings braying porn stars to screeching orgasms at the slightest pelvic thrust—they take a lot more coordination and communication than that to achieve success. But they're great for mutual masturbation with shared penetration, or for putting on masturbation shows for each other while trying to keep the dildo(s) in place. Their extra length makes double dildos excellent for people with limited mobility range. And all doubles, from the classics to the Feeldoe and Nexus, can be enjoyed and used successfully (read: orgasm) by male-female couples.

Your strap-on adventures needn't be limited to the standard variety pubic protuberance. For instance, a thigh harness can make a lap dance or leg ride very rewarding. Thigh harnesses either buckle onto your leg with a nylon strap or slide on via elastic band, and some will come with a dildo already seated in the strap-on. But the best version of this clever device has a hole or O-ring that allows you to change out dildos on a whim. Most of the nylon strap and buckle varieties have very long straps, which are great for big thighs but are often long enough to fit around a waist (pony rides, anyone?), a pillow, a bar stool or piece of furniture that just happens to look at you with a come-hither wink.

A face strap-on is just that: a strap-on apparatus that buckles around the head to seat a dildo either right over the mouth of the wearer, or on the forehead. This type of strap-on effectively makes the wearer's head into a sex toy and provides a hell of a view for the harness wearer. Most have the dildo already attached, but try to find a head harness that allows you to use different dildos interchangeably so you can use a dildo in the size and shape you like and take the dildo out for thorough cleaning.

People with neck or jaw injuries or whose neck muscles might strain easily will want to be a little more physically cautious and establish good communication with the person they're penetrating, as it's easy for someone near orgasm to buck a little too hard, or grab the head and thrust roughly. If you're worried about neck strain, lie on a flat surface with a pillow or two under your neck and head for cushion, or experiment with sex position pillows, like Liberator Shapes (liberatorshapes.com).

Chapter 11

The Art of Pegging

H e tells you he wants it. And you're more than ready to give it to him. Perhaps you have a scenario in mind, a fantasy you'll both act out with the strap-on as the key ingredient. Or maybe you're simply pegging for the sake of it, the feeling, the intimacy, the fun. Just adding it to your routine sexual encounters is delightful.

While pegging lends itself easily to role play and fantasy scenes, it's such a versatile sex act that it can easily be incorporated into your everyday sex lives. No uniforms, dog collars or fake accents necessary—just a guy and a girl, and their strap-on. Or, a strap-on shared by three.

Strap-On Sex à la Carte

But how does it work, exactly? It might seem daunting at first to try and imagine how you'd go from making out and groping and getting hot to—wait a minute, I have to go get this thing on, and oops the buckles aren't working and now I have to get the dildo in place, and do I look funny dancing around with this turquoise dildo in my hand trying to shove it in my pants? Sometimes this might happen—the unintentional sexual silliness that makes sex play, *play*. But if you think ahead a bit, you can have everything ready to go so you slip into your harness in one smooth move, and carry on.

When you get your harness and dildo, take a minute before your hot date to try it on, set the adjustments and get a sense of the "right fit." Clean all your sex toys—butt plugs and dildos—so you know you're ready to play. Get the lube in a handy spot, and any gloves or finger cots you might be planning to use to get him warmed up. If possible, fit the dildo you want to start out with into the harness so you're all set to go when you want to transition from regular sex to adding a strap-on into the mix.

When you're both hot and ready to play, you can switch activities and get your strap-on on in whatever way makes you feel sexiest. You can pause the activities and daringly stand up, keep eye contact with your lover and wickedly slip into the harness. You could make him fetch it for you, and erotically command him to help you put it on. Or a surprise might be in order, one where you're already wearing the harness under your clothing, and at the right moment you reach into the side table and present him with your intentions.

Then, back to making out, making love, sixty-nining—whatever you were doing before, but with a new toy for him to play with. Let him—or make him—explore it with his hands, or even his mouth. Lube it up and put it in his hand and see what he does with it—often, this is a very revealing move, and you can observe the sort of movements with which he usually touches his *own* cock. Rub your penises together, or even put his thighs together and fuck the space in between.

Strap-On Sex and Role Play

If you choose to go the fantasy route for framing your strap-on encounters, you have pretty much every fantasy involving a dick (or two, if you include his) to choose from. Scenarios for strap-on sex can range from hot and heavy dominatrix scenes where you make him your slave and he has to worship and submit to your cock, to fetish scenes of pony play, all the way to gender swaps or even "sailors trapped on a ship."

If you're role-playing with a strap-on, consider these ideas:

- A doctor or nurse scene, where the male patient might need to get his temperature taken in an unconventional way, or may require unusual treatments.
- A classic male environment that becomes sexual, such as an encounter in a locker room, at football practice, in a military barracks, on sailing ships, or any other all-male enclave.
- Fetishy scenes that involve human animals (like dogs, ponies, or other animals, like tigers).
- A police scene with a surprise nightstick.
- A prostitution scenario, with varying gender roles.
- Gender play where you reverse gender roles and he becomes a female character and has to "learn the ropes" as a woman.

When you suck strap-on cock, you're putting on a show.

For Him: How to Go Down on a Strap-On

One look at your lover in a sexy harness, all buckles and straps, with an erect member jutting suggestively from her body, and it's difficult to resist the temptation to swallow her whole. What's great about sucking her strap-on is that not only does she get a hot show to watch, but the pressure at the dildo's base is directly over her clit—so you know you're making her feel good, too. Many of the same principles, tricks, and skills apply to fellating a dildo on your lover as do to going down on an actual cock; you'll want to do what you like, what you know feels good to you, and what you'd like her to do to you—after all, she'll be watching and likely taking notes. But the important difference in giving head to a strap-on is that you will approach the techniques you apply from a different angle: instead of being focused on the way the penis *feels*, you're focused on how the owner *sees* you.

Just before entry, you'll want to be sure that his penis is being stimulated.

When you suck strap-on cock, you're putting on a show, and making the wearer feel hot in that harness—and it's probably a big turn-on for you, too. See how you treat the dildo visually, and maintain plenty of eye contact, employ very visual oral techniques, and use your hands a lot. Your hands can roam, jerk the dildo off in your face, or grab her hips to pull her into you, or you can stimulate her beneath the harness with your fingers—though she might want to do this herself. The way you give head to a dildo is different for the reasons I just mentioned, but strap-on fellatio is also unique in that you aren't necessarily giving a blowjob that ends with an orgasm. You're down there until you or she decides you're finished, or you both decide to switch activities.

Getting It On

Hot and bothered, lubed up, warmed up, hungry for pegging—penetration is what's for breakfast. Just as if you were inserting a finger for the first time, coat your dildo with copious amounts of lube and apply lubricant to his anus (cold lube is a shock—warm it in your hand first). Tease your finger in and out so you know he's good and ready, and then move forward with your dildo so the tip is just at his opening. At this point, just before entry, you'll want to be sure that his penis is being stimulated, either by your hand or his. You may have to take your hand off his cock to steady yourself for a slow, smooth entry, but try to keep him stimulated as steadily as possible throughout your initial penetration. This will make the experience much more pleasurable for him than otherwise.

Gently, slowly ease into him. Move the dildo in an inch, maybe two, and pause. Let his muscles adjust around the dildo, and let the muscles relax and pull the tip of your dildo in. Once in, move forward a little bit and wait another second. Then ask him how it feels, and what he wants you to do next.

> Gently, slowly ease into him. Move the dildo in an inch, maybe two, and pause.

If all systems are go but he's totally given up control to you for the next moves, then proceed to slowly move in and out of him, maintaining the stimulation to his penis. Reapply lube frequently, even if it's everywhere and you don't think he needs it. Be absolutely careful about not using the anally lubed hand for contact with your vagina, or anything you don't want bacteria on or in. You can choose to stop playing with him and just get into thrusting—watch his body language and check in with him before you change speed, depth or intensity of your thrusting. When in doubt, hold perfectly still with your dildo in his ass and tell him to set the pace. As he nears orgasm, pay attention to the way you're thrusting, and keep the same pace until orgasm. These could be deep, long, slow strokes, or hard, fast bucks—or somewhere in between.

How to Come in a Harness

How will you come yourself while pleasuring your lover with a strap-on? Here are a few recommendations for getting off while in your harness.

- Masturbate.
- Slip on a finger vibe and rub your clit.
- Slide a bullet vibe into the harness.
- Look for a "coupler" sleeve at sex shops that attaches to the harness to hold a dildo inside you.
- Slip into a wearable vibrator before you don your harness. Take turns with the controls.

Penetration Techniques and Positions

You'll find and develop your own "best practices" as you go along, but here are a few suggestions to get you started.

- Have him show you how he likes to jack off—with your dildo.
- Get a sloppy blowjob.
- Rub your penis all over his face.
- Lube up and fuck different crevices all over his body.
- Lube up both of your cocks and rub them together.
- Try penetrating him in all the positions you've enjoyed up till now: sixty-nine, missionary position, doggy-style, "man on top."
- Make out while your dicks touch.
- Let him "discover" it in your pants or under your skirt.

Fun Things to Do When You're Fucking Him

What's a favorite recipe without the garnish? Here are a few spicy toppings.

- Pinch his nipples.
- Kiss him, intensely.
- Tell him how sexy he looks.
- Jack him off with each thrust.
- Spank his ass.
- Make him suck your fingers or nipples—or a dildo.
- Have him jack himself off while you fuck him.

Afterward, you'll probably both be locked in a position that has you still inside him, and him a melted puddle of orgasmically blissed-out butter. Take control and have him take a few deep breaths as you pull out of him—it will be a very intense feeling, so you want to go slow. Three deep breaths are a fine idea; pull out a little on each exhale, and all the way out on his final one. Be sure to move the dildo away from everything—it has bacteria on it, so behave accordingly. Slide out of your harness and set it aside or take it to a cleaning area; hand him a towel or baby wipes or suggest that you shower together. Most of all, right after you peg—cuddle. Kiss. Smile.

Tips for Adding a Third Partner

If, as discussed in chapter 7, you and your lover decide to make room in your harness play for a third party, aim for having a variety of sex toys at hand, and always plenty of lubricant. Vibrators can keep your arousal level high when you're not being directly stimulated, or one of you can masturbate while watching the other being pegged. A butt plug can be set in place for hands-free anal stimulation, and there are arrays of vibrators available that can be worn like panties; some are even operated by remote control. Just be sure to follow cleanliness guidelines for sharing toys. Dildos and harnesses can make a threesome seem like an orgy. The combinations are as endless as your imagination.

> Dildos and harnesses can make a threesome seem like an orgy.

Sex Positions for Three and a Harness

You can do a lot with several bodies, and the potential for pleasure is limitless. Here are ideas for harness play for a threesome.

- Team up and perform oral sex together on the third; especially if she's wearing the harness.

- Use your hands to masturbate the harness wearer while the third one licks his or her genitals.
- Hold the second person on your lap (facing outward), with both of your legs spread, while the third performs oral sex on that person's dildo; or, the third wears the harness and penetrates the person on your lap.
- Try face-sitting while the harness wearer penetrates the person beneath you.
- Put the third person on all fours while one licks or penetrates his or her genitals (with a harness) and the other enjoys his or her mouth (or gets a strap-on blowjob).
- Make a "sandwich" out of someone by putting him or her in the middle. With a man in the middle, he can penetrate one partner while being penetrated by another's fingers, penis or dildo. With a woman in the middle, she can be penetrated while penetrating another with her strap-on.
- One can always simply fuck the second with a strap-on while the third performs oral sex on—either!
- Lick or fellate in a daisy chain of oral sex.

The Secret

Alison Tyler

JACKSON AND I have a special place where we picnic. It's at the top of a small hill on the very edge of the Castro. From our vantage point we can see tennis courts and apartment buildings, many with rainbow flags fluttering from the balconies. Generally, we spread out a blanket, pull the cork on a bottle of wine, and kick back, gazing at the multicolored dragon kites fluttering overhead.

The first time we went up to the hill was for a punishment session. I had a heavy belt on that day, and I took Jackson up with me and forced him to hold on to a nearby chain-link fence with both hands. I reached around his waist and undid his brown Dickies, sliding them down his muscular thighs to reveal his amazing ass. He never wears underwear—neither boxers nor briefs—which made my job of smacking his delicious rear with my belt that much easier. I chose a time when there was little foot traffic, and I don't believe anyone saw or heard us. It doesn't take that long to get in a good twelve strokes. Still, even if someone had caught the tail end, so to speak, we wouldn't have been bothered. People are pretty relaxed about those sorts of things in this part of San Francisco.

That was then.

This time, I had other ideas. I told my six-foot-tall, handsome brown-eyed man to wear a pair of drawstring pants, knowing he'd go bare beneath as usual. He paired a cobalt blue

T-shirt with the pants, and a formfitting cashmere sweater I'd bought him last Valentine's Day. I had on a ribbed white tank top and denim jacket, and my dark blonde hair hung straight and loose down my back. But under my favorite pair of well-worn jeans was the real treat...the surprise I could hardly manage to keep secret. Every few seconds on the drive over, I opened my mouth to tell him...but somehow, I managed to remain silent.

When we got to our spot, I spread out the blanket on the soft carpet of grass. Jackson got comfortable, stretching out his long legs, crossing his arms under his head. I bent to kiss him before climbing on top of him, straddling him so that he could feel. Since we'd first discussed coming here on this day, I'd been dying to reveal my plans. But now I was glad I'd waited.

"Oh, god," Jackson sighed when he felt me against him. "You're packing, Dana, aren't you?"

I just smiled.

My wallet was chained to my belt loops, and I considered lassoing that chain around his wrists. Jackson likes the feel of metal against his skin. He craves being under my control. But I thought better of it, leaning over to pull a blindfold from the picnic basket, like a magician performing a trick.

Jackson tilted his face toward mine automatically, letting me fasten the blindfold in place without a word.

"Can anyone see?" he asked softly.

"The question is, can *you* see?" I asked right back.

He shook his head. "But can anyone see me?" I smiled and looked around. We had spread our old green army blanket beneath a tree off to the side of the walking path. Way at the bottom, two young men were talking, both with small dogs on leashes. No one else was in sight. Instead of answering his query,

I slid down his body and pressed my lips to Jackson's cock through his thin black pants and whispered, "Just me."

He sighed at the feel of my words vibrating through the material and against his skin. Then he lifted his hips, pressing toward my hungry mouth, and I grinned and licked him through the light cotton. I know what my lover likes most. He craves the danger of being caught and the excitement of having things done to him in public, with the sun beating down on him and the prospect of curious eyes upon him.

As I slowly pulled down his pants, I began telling him stories, the things he most likes to hear. I said, "Jackson, now I think I see someone. Two women walking this way."

It was a harmless fabrication.

Or, rather, a total lie.

No one was even close to spotting us, but Jackson moaned softly when he heard me, imagining the scenario better than I could ever describe it. People watching him. People *seeing*.

I sat at his side, wrapping one of my fists around his cock, making him shudder as I continued my fib. "They're looking at you," I said, softly. "They want to see me suck you. Can I let them watch, baby? Can I let them watch me suck your cock?"

Jackson murmured "Yes," and I bent to lick along the length of his erection, to drag my tongue along the shaft, to roll the metal ball that pierces my tongue over and over his sensitive tip. Then I sat upright again, saying, "They were totally shocked. They kept walking."

Jackson grinned widely. He liked that.

Now I had him roll over on the blanket. I sucked one finger into my mouth, getting it nice and wet, and then skated my moistened fingertip around his asshole. My man groaned once more, darker this time, louder. Without hesitation, I gently slipped the finger inside of him. I could tell that he couldn't believe I was doing that here. In public. But I didn't care.

"Oh, fucking god," Jackson murmured.

I reached into the picnic basket with my free hand, rummaging for the lube I'd brought with me. Slowly, I poured a bit of the clear liquid down the split between Jackson's cheeks. Then I added another finger, feeling my man clench down on me. I was sitting with one leg crossed under my body, and I rocked forward, pressing my pussy against my heel. Touching Jackson like this turned him on, sure. But it drove me crazy with desire, as well. Gradually, I worked until I had pushed three fingers inside him, my digits heavy with silver rings. He clenched his cheeks, tightening his hole in response to the way I was treating him.

And now I continued with my script.

"Someone else is coming," I said, thinking that I was going to be coming soon. I just love to play with Jackson's fine ass. Nothing excites me more. Well, nothing except what I was planning to do next.

"I'm going to fuck you, now," I hissed in his ear.

He squirmed, unsure, but I didn't hesitate. I removed my fingers and parted the cheeks of his ass. The spring breeze had a bite in it, and I knew Jackson could feel the cool rush against his most private place. Quickly, I lubed him up more, loving the way his body responded to my touch. Now Jackson stiffened, in doubt about what I was going to do, obviously unsure whether I would actually go through with what I'd told him, but wishing desperately that I would.

There was no one anywhere near us, and I undid my slacks and oiled up my dark pink cock before climbing on top of him.

Jackson whispered anxiously, "Is someone watching?"

I pushed the head of my toy inside of my man, and he groaned, but he kept talking. "Dana, is anyone watching? Tell me."

I thrust the dildo into his ass and leaned forward, talking low and soft in his ear as I began to do push-ups on him, fucking his ass in the perfect rhythm. I had a difficult time finding the words, my breath was coming fast and ragged, but I managed for Jackson's sake. The story I was telling him excited my man as much as the workout I was giving his ass. "Yeah, Jackson," I said, quickly. "Yeah, Jackson. Four of 'em. Four women at the edge of the path are looking our way. They're watching you get that cute asshole of yours reamed. I'll bet they're wishing they could line up and take turns."

He moaned and then stiffened as I continued to drive into him, continued to fuck that tight rosebud opening I like so much. He craves to be taken in this manner, roughly, in public, exposed.

"You'd like that, wouldn't you? You'd like to be their toy. To have each one oil up your asshole, drive inside of you with a different cock. Each one bigger than the last. It would be a veritable gang bang, baby. First me, then one stranger after another. But you know what?"

"What?" he panted. "What, Dana?"

"I'd take a final turn at the end. I'd be the one to make you come."

"Oh, god," he sighed, and I could tell he was close. "Oh, god, Dana."

I pounded even harder now, and I reached one hand under his body and gripped his cock. I pulled on him, tugging as I continued to fuck him, and when he came, I came right after, so that we were a mess of sweet sex juices and slippery lube, my hand coated, our blanket stained. And none of that bothering me a bit.

When I heard real voices—not the imaginary ones I'd concocted for my love—I hurried up and pulled out, tucking my soiled cock into my jeans and covering Jackson with the blanket. Quickly, I undid the blindfold as Jackson hiked up his pants. He rolled over and sat up, brushing his long hair out of his eyes, helping me put away our equipment.

"No one was there, right?" he asked as we made our way back to the parking lot.

I shrugged. I know when to keep a secret.

Chapter 12

Shopping and Further Study

Strap-on play requires the right gear; the trick is finding what you want in a well-made package—and actually having that package arrive, with your privacy intact. Many sex toys found at garden-variety retail outlets are poorly made, some retailers don't care if you get a broken toy, and every online shopper needs to be careful about privacy issues. Even if your credit card is insured against fraud and the site uses a secure ordering database, you'll still need to make sure you didn't get on an unwanted email list or are otherwise violated in the process.

Window-shop to get ideas before you dig out the credit card; you may get inspired by seeing toys you didn't know existed. If you just want some fantasy fodder, browse through a retailer's toys (do this together, it's quite fun), whether online or at a physical store. Couples who shop together will discover that shopping is its own foreplay, and even the online ordering process can result in a quickie at the computer. But what's really great about shopping for sex toys together is making new

discoveries about things you'd each like to try, and in the bar-
gain learning a lot about each other.

First decide what it is you hope to accomplish (strap-on sex,
an adventure with a vibrating butt plug, finding the right lube)
then find the place that has your item. Chances are high, however, that you'll wind up shopping at more than one retailer
to get everything you want—sadly, no one has it all.
Unfortunately, most big sex toy retailers have exclusive agree-
ments with distributors or manufacturers that make it tough
for a consumer to find all the toys he or she wants at only one
store. The big retailers have lots of poorly made stuff, while
the boutiques have high-quality products yet will charge you
an arm and a leg for lube you can get cheaper elsewhere (like
Amazon). Amazon, too, has its disadvantages as you'll still have
your items shipped from different warehouses within the
Amazon empire (meaning various arrival times for your packages), and the quality will vary greatly from store to store. And
don't expect these stores to have great return policies on broken
items.

Most people buy their sex toys online. Online privacy and
security makes it easy and safe for anyone to try out new sexual
ideas and explore new possibilities, and online retailers put sex
toys within everyone's geographic reach. However, the Internet
can be dicey if you don't know the company's privacy policy
(some companies sell your information to other parties), and
it's difficult to ask questions about the products, unless the company provides an information phone line on their site.

When shopping online take every precaution to safeguard
your privacy. Only shop at reputable sites; if you're not sure about
their reputation, see if they have online forums where you can

garner customer feedback, or check to see if they have actual brick-and-mortar stores (a sign of stability), or Google their URL and name to see what you dig up. Look at their privacy policy—if it's dodgy, shop elsewhere. See how they ship their products—is it done discreetly, and do the toys come in plain packages? And finally, see how their products are presented— if they have offensive or misspelled product descriptions or sell products that are unsafe, or if they just seem a bit off, then they'll likely treat their customers with the same disdain. Do they have annoying pop-up windows when you're trying to shop? Skip 'em. Shop with a company you like (vote with your credit card!), and if that company has an educational section or mission statement, even better.

In a real, in-person store, don't go anywhere you feel weird or uncomfortable; it should be no more than a place to shop. Sex toy boutiques are styled specifically toward couples and single women. You'll see a lot of other women (and men) shopping there—people of every stripe and persuasion, having fun buying vibrators and cock rings. Unfortunately these clean, well-lit places to shop for sex toys are found in only a few major cities (see resource lists in the next section).

All major cities have a selection of adult toy, book, and video shops that are somewhat (or even very) sleazy and uncomfortable to shop in, generally because they aren't clean or kept up in any visible way, and the customers and clerks don't seem to want to be there. While these can be a "walk on the wild side" for couples, keep in mind that you'll likely see things in the store that will totally turn you off or offend you—or will make you run from the store laughing. Often, though, these stores are not so scary and you'll get what you want, pay the bored cashier (who's seen it all, by the way), and go home to get it on and get off with your new toys. Either way, it's highly recommended that, before you buy anything online or in person, you make the trek to a store so that you can see and handle the toys in person at least once, giving you both a realistic idea of what you're buying (or not).

Online Shopping in the United States

Adam and Eve: adameve.com

Aneros Prostate Stimulator: aneros.com

A Woman's Touch: a-womans-touch.com (retail store in Madison)

Babeland: babeland.com (retail stores in Seattle, New York and Los Angeles)

Blowfish: blowfish.com

Eve's Garden: evesgarden.com (retail store in New York)

Extreme Restraints: extremerestraints.com

Fatale Media: fatalemedia.com (for the film *Bend Over Boyfriend* and other great sex how-to videos)

Forbidden Fruit: forbiddenfruit.com (retail store in Austin)

Good Vibrations: goodvibes.com (retail stores in San Francisco, Berkeley and Boston)

Hidden Self: hiddenself.com

Hustler Hollywood: hustlerhollywood.com (retail stores in West Hollywood, Gardena, San Diego, Monroe, Cincinnati, Nashville, New Orleans, Lexington and Ft. Lauderdale)

Libida: libida.com

My Pleasure: mypleasure.com

Pleasure Chest: thepleasurechest.com (retail stores in New York, Los Angeles and Chicago)

Purple Passion: purplepassion.com
Sportsheets: sportsheets.com
Tantus Silicone: tantussilicone.com (silicone toys; the Feeldoe)
Vixen Creations: vixencreations.com (silicone toys; Nexus, Nexus
    Jr., VixSkin™)
Xandria: xandria.com

Online Shopping in Canada

Come As You Are: comeasyouare.com (retail store in Toronto)
Good for Her: goodforher.com (retail store in Toronto)
Lovecraft: lovecraftsexshop.com
Womyn's Ware: womynsware.com (retail store in Vancouver)

Online Shopping in the United Kingdom

Ann Summers: annsummers.com
Babes 'N Horny: babes-n-horny.com
Blissbox: blissbox.com
Cliterati: cliteratishop.co.uk
Coco de Mer: coco-de-mer.co.uk (retail store in Covent Garden,
    London)
Hustler Hollywood: hustlerhollywood.co.uk
LoveHoney: lovehoney.co.uk
Loving Angles: loving-angles.com
Myla: myla.com (retail stores in Notting Hill and South
    Kensington, London)
Sh! Women's Erotic Emporium: sh-womenstore.com (retail store in
    Shoreditch, London)
Taboo: taboo.co.uk

Online Shopping in Australia and New Zealand

bliss4women.com (retail store in Melbourne)

D.vice: dvice.co.nz (retail stores in Auckland, Wellington, Melbourne and Palmerston North)

Femplay: femplay.com.au

Ms. Naughty's for the Girls Superstore: store.sex-superstore.com

Sharon Austen: sharonausten.com.au

Online Shopping in Europe

Blissbox: blissbox.com (sites for shipping to Netherlands, Germany, Belgium)

Concorde Boutique: concorde.fr (retail store in Paris)

Demonia: demonia.com (retail store in Paris)

Fleshion: fleshion.com (France)

Sexou: sexou.com (France)

Voissa: voissa.com (France)

More Online Resources

Aneros Prostate Massage, aneros.com

Pegging: Wikipedia, en.wikipedia.org/wiki/Pegging_(sexual_practice)

Prostate Massage: Wikipedia, en.wikipedia.org/wiki/Prostate_massage

Prostate: Wikipedia, en.wikipedia.org/wiki/Prostate

Highly Recommended Reading

The Guide to Getting It On! by Paul Joannides

Men's Private Parts: An Owner's Manual by James H. Gilbaugh, MD

The New Male Sexuality: The Truth About Men, Sex and Pleasure by
   Bernie Zilbergeld, PhD

Nina Hartley's Guide to Total Sex by Nina Hartley with I.S. Levine

The Sexual Male: Problems and Solutions by Richard Milsten, MD,
   and Julian Slowinski, PsyD

*The Survivor's Guide to Sex: How to Have an Empowered Sex Life After
   Child Sexual Abuse* by Staci Haines

Tricks to Please a Man Jay Wiseman

The Ultimate Guide to Anal Sex for Men by Bill Brent

The Ultimate Guide to Anal Sex for Women by Tristan Taormino

The Ultimate Guide to Cunnilingus by Violet Blue

The Ultimate Guide to Sex and Disability by Miriam Kaufman, Cory
   Silverberg and Fran Odette

The Ultimate Guide to Sexual Fantasy by Violet Blue

The Ultimate Guide to Strap-On Sex by Karlyn Lotney

Strap-On Porn

(A caveat: it's difficult to find respectful videos on this topic.)

Babes Ballin' Boys, low-budget series, Pleasure Productions

Bend Over Boyfriend 1 and *2*, Fatale Media and SIR Productions

The Opening of Misty Beethoven, VCA

Slide Bi Me, Sexpositive Productions

Strap Attack, Strap Attack 2, Evil Angel (very intense, advanced players)

Strapon Chicks #15: Stick it to the Man, Ducati Productions (high
   recommendation)

The Ultimate Guide to Anal Sex for Women #2, Evil Angel

Bisexual movies with porn star Tina Tyler in them, such as *Biagra*
   and *Fine Bi Me*

Safe Sex Info

Before you put each other's naughty bits in your mouths or even think about rubbing your bodies together, it's a good idea to know where these bits have been. But since we don't all live in a perfect world—in fact, no one does—you'll want to use condoms, gloves, dental dams or finger cots when you have oral, vaginal and anal sex; when you use or share sex toys; and in some cases, when you give hand jobs. When someone pulls out a condom, dam glove or 'cot, you know you're in good hands. Here are the items in your first line of defense against invading infections and viruses, in short order:

Condoms: Available in latex and polyurethane, in dozens of sizes, colors and flavors. Animal skin condoms do not prevent the spread of some viruses. A condom is a snug sheath that unrolls onto a penis or sex toy. Use condoms for fellatio, vaginal and anal sex, for covering sex toys that are made of porous materials, or for when you want to share a sex toy. Change condoms for different sex partners and orifices—something used anally should be covered with a new condom before being inserted orally or vaginally. Don't reuse your toy condoms. Do not use anything containing oils of any kind where latex condoms may come in contact; however, polyurethane condoms may be used with oils.

Dental Dams: Thin squares of latex or polyurethane used as barriers for cunnilingus and rimming. Lubricate the genitals, place the dam on top, keep a good hold on the dam and lick to your heart's content. Available in a few flavors and colors. In a jam you can use plastic wrap or a condom cut open and laid flat.

Gloves: Use latex or nonlatex gloves for hand jobs on any gender. They protect against germs from your hands going onto genitals, can protect your hands from picking up viruses or germs, and make hands a smooth surface free of jagged nails or scratchy calluses.

Finger Cots: Tiny condoms made of latex that unroll over a finger to create a sterile surface. Great for on-the-go escapades.

If you choose to go at it uncovered, here is what you are at risk for. Make an informed decision!

Sharing Sex Toys

HIGH RISK	MODERATE RISK	NO RISK	N/A
Chlamydia	Bacterial vaginosis	None	None
Gonorrhea	Hepatitis A		
Hepatitis B	Hepatitis C		
HIV	Herpes		
Syphilis	HPV		
	Lice/scabies		
	Vaginitis		

Anal to Oral Contact (Penis or Sex Toy)

HIGH RISK	MODERATE RISK	NO RISK	N/A
Gonorrhea	HIV	Lice/scabies	Bacterial vaginosis
Hepatitis A	Chlamydia		Vaginitis
Hepatitis B	Hepatitis C		
Herpes			
HPV			
Syphilis			

Unprotected Anal to Vaginal Contact

HIGH RISK	MODERATE RISK	NO RISK	N/A
Bacterial vaginosis	Hepatitis C		Lice/scabies
Chlamydia			
Gonorrhea			
Hepatitis A			
Hepatitis B			
Herpes			
HIV			
HPV			
Syphilis			

Unprotected Rimming (Getting)

HIGH RISK	MODERATE RISK	NO RISK	N/A
High Risk	Moderate Risk	No Risk	N/A
Gonorrhea	Chlamydia	Hepatitis A	Bacterial vaginosis
Hepatitis B	Hepatitis C		Vaginitis
Herpes	HPV		
Syphilis	HIV		
	Lice/scabies		

Unprotected Rimming (Giving)

HIGH RISK	MODERATE RISK	NO RISK	N/A
Gonorrhea	Chlamydia		Bacterial vaginosis
Hepatitis A	Hepatitis C		Vaginitis
Hepatitis B	HIV		
Herpes	Lice/scabies		
HPV			
Syphilis			

About the Author

VIOLET BLUE is the best-selling, award-winning author and editor of over a dozen books on sex and sexuality, including *The Smart Girl's Guide to Porn*, *The Ultimate Guide to Cunnilingus*, and *The Ultimate Guide to Fellatio*, all available from Cleis Press (www.cleispress.com). Violet is a sex educator who lectures at University of California branches and community teaching institutions, and writes about erotica, pornography, sexual pleasure and health. She is a professional sex blogger and femmebot; the sex columnist for the *San Francisco Chronicle*; an author at Metroblogging San Francisco; and is on the Gawker Media payroll at Fleshbot. She is a San Francisco native and human blog; she lists her profession as "wetware hacker" and her sexual orientation as binary. She has survived being a Dorkbot presenter twice and over ten years at Survival Research Laboratories, and is a notorious podcaster and videoblogger. Her podcast Open Source Sex has made iTunes cry for its mommy at least once. She has been interviewed, featured, and quoted as an expert by more magazine, web, television, and radio outlets than can be listed here, including Boing Boing, the *Wall Street Journal*, *Newsweek*, NPR, MSNBC, CNN, *Wired*, *Esquire* and Web MD; for more information visit her websites tinynibbles.com and techyum.com, or listen to her podcast, Open Source Sex.

Printed in the United States
By Bookmasters